35

W9-CKI-367

Medical Illuminations

MEDICAL ILLUMINATIONS

*Using Evidence, Visualization
and Statistical Thinking to Improve
Healthcare*

HOWARD WAINER
National Board of Medical Examiners

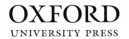
OXFORD
UNIVERSITY PRESS

OXFORD

UNIVERSITY PRESS

Great Clarendon Street, Oxford, OX2 6DP,
United Kingdom

Oxford University Press is a department of the University of Oxford.
It furthers the University's objective of excellence in research, scholarship,
and education by publishing worldwide. Oxford is a registered trade mark of
Oxford University Press in the UK and in certain other countries

Published in the United States of America by Oxford University Press
198 Madison Avenue, New York, NY 10016, United States of America

British Library Cataloguing in Publication Data
Data available

Library of Congress Control Number: 2013938497

ISBN 978–0–19–966879–3

Printed in the UK by
Bell & Bain Ltd, Glasgow

Oxford University Press makes no representation, express or implied, that the
drug dosages in this book are correct. Readers must therefore always check
the product information and clinical procedures with the most up-to-date
published product information and data sheets provided by the manufacturers
and the most recent codes of conduct and safety regulations. The authors and
the publishers do not accept responsibility or legal liability for any errors in the
text or for the misuse or misapplication of material in this work. Except where
otherwise stated, drug dosages and recommendations are for the non-pregnant
adult who is not breast-feeding

Links to third party websites are provided by Oxford in good faith and
for information only. Oxford disclaims any responsibility for the materials
contained in any third party website referenced in this work.

Dedication

To the Yankees:
From Yogi, Mickey and Scooter,
To Derek, Jorge and Mo.
Sixty Years of Evidence

PREFACE

It is rare to find apostasy on the staid and dignified pages of *The New York Times*, and yet there it was, not once, but twice, prominently displayed in the Sunday Review section on June 3, 2012.

On the first page, above the fold, was an article by Elizabeth Rosenthal MD, "Let's (not) get physicals," in which she lays out the evidence against the almost canonized ritual of an annual physical exam. She points out that, "For decades, scientific research has shown that annual physical exams—and many of the screening tests that routinely accompany them—are in many ways pointless or (worse) dangerous, because they can lead to unneeded procedures." She then goes on to list ten routine screening tests and medical procedures that research indicates ought to be jettisoned.

After recovering my breath I turned to the inside of the section to read the continuation of Dr. Rosenthal's article, only to be greeted by a second essay, by Gary Taubes, a medical researcher at the Robert Wood Johnson Foundation, explaining that evidence suggests that eating less salt can sometimes worsen our health!

As I read these two remarkable reports I flashed back to a line in Woody Allen's 1973 film "Sleeper" in which Miles Monroe, the lead character, after awaking from a two centuries long nap, is offered a cigarette and told "don't worry, it's <u>real</u> tobacco; it's good for you, like malteds and bacon."

What happened to turn accepted medical wisdom on its head? The short answer is "evidence." But as evidence accrues to provide a convincing argument for changing medical practice, another question emerges: if this evidence has been around for so long, why has it taken until now for the suggestion that we change practice? And, now that these results, garnered from scientific journals, have progressed far enough to find themselves in the popular media, why are there still staunch defenders of the status quo?

These puzzles, exemplified in these two recent articles, are what piqued my curiosity over the past few years and led to this book. In it I take a case-study approach to explore a number of medical situations spanning the evaluation of hip fractures, the value of mammograms, and the use of glucose meters to help control diabetes. In the course of telling these stories I recognized that sometimes we have to go a little out of the way in order to come back a short distance correctly.[1] And so the beginning of the book is a detour that examines both why it is important for the medical care consuming public to understand often-subtle evidence and how we might communicate that evidence better. One important part of the answer to this are graphical displays. Surprisingly, I continue this tale by introducing Will Burtin, a remarkable refugee from Nazi Germany, who came to this country with little English but possessed of an extraordinary ability to communicate complex material in pictures. He spent much of his long career working in medicine and a single graph that he produced provides the raw material for a running start into my narrative.

But there would be no narrative at all without the cooperation and advice I received from a fairly large number of my colleagues. It is my honor and my pleasure to express gratitude to them now.

First, let me begin with Donald Melnick, president of the National Board of Medical Examiners, whose leadership provides the resources, atmosphere and encouragement for scholars to pursue extended projects like this one. He also, when asked, dipped into his impressive medical memory to offer suggestions about possibly fruitful paths. Next, my thanks to Ron Nungester and Brian Clauser, who read everything that appears here, and much that, happily, does not. They also provided time and quiet.

Also, my gratitude to my collaborators on much of the work that was synthesized into this book. I begin with my coauthors: Peter Baldwin, Joseph Bernstein, Michael Larsen, Shaun Lysen, Sam Savage and Paul Velleman. Next, I must thank colleagues and friends who offered crucial help all along the way: Steve Clyman, David Donoho, Bob Galbraith, Kyung Han, David Hoaglin, Peter Scoles and Xiaohui Wang. Chapter 2 would have been very barren indeed without the contributions of Jana Asher, Georgette Asherman, Jacques Bertin, Troy Brandt, Mindy Chang, Pierre Dangauthier, Céline Dartois, Lawrence B. Finer, Dibyojyoti Haldar, Benjamin and Katherine Lauderdale, Mark Nicolich, Philip Price, Christian C. Ryan, Brian and Christine Schmotzer, Donald Schopflocher and Justin Talbot.

Of course, I would never get anything done without the help and supervision of Editha Chase, who takes care of everything; doing it so quickly and perfectly.

Special thanks to Drs. Marc Drimmer and Rachel Dultz for restoring to me a treasure most dear.

Profound contributions are sometimes hard to pinpoint. My wife, Linda Steinberg, reads far more widely than I do and tells me of many wonderful ideas and facts that she has harvested. Her judgment has always been remarkable and what I was able to retrieve from our conversations has enriched this story in too many ways to recount. She also reads much of what I have written and her suggestions have improved clarity and grammar, while subtracting pomposity. I thank her for all of this; and for her permission to keep in some of the semicolons.

Last, my thanks to the editorial and production staff of Oxford University Press whose professional expertise helped me to more nearly say what I meant. Primus inter pares among the many who added their professional expertise are: Clare Charles, Gandhimathi Ganesan, Claire Hopwood, Keith Mansfield, Victoria Mortimer and Penny Sucharov.

Howard Wainer
Pennington, NJ
April 2013

CONTENTS

Annotated Contents   *xiii*

Introduction   1

SECTION I—COMMUNICATING WITH THE PUBLIC

1. New York's cancer maps: What we don't know won't hurt us,
   it's what we do know that ain't   9

2. A centenary celebration for Will Burtin: A pioneer
   of scientific visualization   21

3. That's funny . . .   50

4. Commentary on some graphs in the *2008 National Healthcare
   Quality Report*   59

5. Improving graphic displays by controlling creativity   74

SECTION II—SOME ADVANCES

6. Diabetes and the obesity epidemic: Taking a better look
   at blood sugar as a start   87

7. A second look at second opinions, with hip fractures
   as an example   99

8. False positives or is a pound of prevention worth
   an ounce of cure   105

9. Assessing long-term risk with shorter-term data   117

10. A remarkable horse: An inquiry into the accuracy
      of medical predictions   122

11. On the role of replication in the advance of science:
      The survival of the fittist   127

SECTION III—ANOTHER HINDRANCE TO PROGRESS

12. What does it take to change practice?   135

13. Why is a raven like a writing desk? Musing on the power
      of convention   145

      Afterword   152

      Notes   *155*
      Bibliography   *166*
      Index   *171*

ANNOTATED CONTENTS

Section I—Communicating with the Public

Chapter 1. New York's cancer maps—The May 11, 2010 issue of the *New York Times* contained an article by Danny Hakim describing legislation sponsored by Assemblyman Richard Brodsky mandating that New York State make public maps showing the incidence of cancer by census tracts throughout the state. Apparently this legislation was passed over the objection of the Health Department. Why would the Health Department object to the public being able to see exactly what was going on? It was reported that both the Health Department and the American Cancer Society felt that the raw data could easily be misunderstood without considerable additional information. This caveat apparently could not deter the legislature. Too bad, it should have. In this chapter I show why.

Chapter 2. A centenary celebration for Will Burtin. Burtin, a pioneer of scientific visualization, immigrated to the United States in 1938 and, in 1951, provided a graphic display of the effects of three new antibiotics on 16 different bacterial infections. His data set provides the grist for opening our eyes to the possibilities. There is no right way to display data, although there are many wrong ways. We take Burtin's data and display it in 16 different ways, commenting on the advantages and disadvantages of each approach and so illustrating why we sometimes require multiple views of the same information to fully comprehend them.

Chapter 3. That's funny . . . Isaac Asimov observed that scientific breakthroughs are rarely accompanied by a cry of "Eureka," much more often one hears "that's funny." The greatest value of a data display is when it <u>forces</u> us to see what we never expected. In this chapter we explore something funny that emerged from some of the displays in Chapter 2. In so doing we discover two results that were only found decades after Burtin's display was published. We speculate that had the data been displayed properly and looked at with an appropriately quizzical mind, the misclassifications of 1951 would have been corrected far sooner.

Chapter 4. Commentary on some graphs in the *2008 National Healthcare Quality Report*. Many national reports are not as polished as they might be. Too often the scientists tasked with preparing the report view Internal Revenue publications as a model of clarity and completeness. In this chapter I look at a recent report and suggest some pathways toward improvement.

Chapter 5. Improving graphic displays by controlling creativity. There is a constant tension in graphic design between new, innovative designs and older, imperfect, but well understood figurations. In this chapter I discuss some graphical solutions to communication problems and try to assess whether the value of an innovative solution is great enough to overcome the comfort and ease of a conventional one. The principal subject of this chapter is the Center for Disease Control's *Atlas of Mortality*, which in many ways should be a model for others to follow.

Section II—Some Advances

Chapter 6. Diabetes and the obesity epidemic. It is estimated that 7% of the population of the United States have diabetes. Coupling the fact that the disease must be managed 24 hours a day, 365 days a year with the average diabetic seeing a health professional only 2–3 hours a year, it stands to reason that the success of disease management depends crucially on the patient. The glucose meter is the principal tool used to monitor the success of the treatment, yet it is designed primarily for the physician's needs and less so for the needs of the patient. In this chapter I describe how the analysis and display of the data collected by the meter can be modified to serve both purposes better. Last I also suggest how the timely feedback on improvident eating from devices likes these can be effective in weight control.

Chapter 7. A second look at second opinions, with hip fractures as an example. In the United States the same story is repeated more than 250,000 times every year. A patient is brought into an emergency room in great pain and is diagnosed quickly with a broken hip. There are two surgical options—pin the fracture (a minor, inexpensive surgery, with a short recovery time) or replace the hip (a major, expensive surgery requiring extensive recuperation). Typically, a surgeon reviews radiographs of the fracture and renders an opinion about which option must be chosen. There is little opportunity for a second opinion. In this chapter we describe a way for the patient to use existing data to improve the surgeon's judgment.

Chapter 8. False positives or is a pound of prevention worth an ounce of cure. Widespread medical screening has the anomalous effect of making the results of the screening almost useless for their intended purpose. We illustrate this with data on mammograms for the detection of breast cancer, PSAs for the detection of prostate cancer, and then expand the argument to show why recent DNA results have revealed surprisingly many imprisoned innocents. We also show why widespread wiretapping to catch terrorists is a deeply flawed strategy.

Chapter 9. Assessing long-term risk with shorter-term data. Drug trials typically take place over two or three years, but once approved those same drugs may be used for decades. In this chapter we explore two approaches for estimating long-term effects from short-term data using the engineering method of accelerated life-testing and the method of low-dose extrapolation pioneered in Delaney Clause research critical in detecting carcinogenic effects of food additives.

Chapter 10. A remarkable horse. Medical predictions, especially in psychiatry, are notoriously unreliable. In this chapter we look at the astounding result reported by the American Psychiatric Association, that psychiatrists' predictions of criminals' future likelihood of recidivism are wrong two-thirds of the time. We discover that this is neither completely true nor all that bad, even when it is true.

Chapter 11. On the role of replication in the advance of science. Promising research results in almost all fields, medicine being no exception, have the annoying property of becoming less promising upon replication. The cause of this troubling result seems to be largely Occidental, for it does not show up in Chinese medical research. In this chapter we explore the phenomenon and hypothesize some plausible causes.

Section III—Another Hindrance to Progress

Chapter 12. What does it take to change practice? Going back to my initial example of Galen's conception of the human uterus this chapter examines a recent breakthrough in improving patient care—a check-list—and compares the adoption of an earlier breakthrough—hand washing—with a pessimistic outlook.

Chapter 13. Why is a raven like a writing desk? Musing on the power of convention. The pie chart, the QWERTY keyboard and written Korean have all existed for a long time, from decades to centuries. During that time suggestions have been made on how to improve them and evidence supporting their efficacy provided. Yet the power of convention has proved to be hard to overcome. In this chapter we examine these three examples in detail.

Introduction

Modern science is complex. It is a mountain whose altitude is composed of arcane methods, specialized vocabulary and advanced mathematics. The common asceticism of mathematical methods provides a kind of unity, but it also separates it from the regions where most people live. For some sciences this isolation is not an insurmountable obstacle to continued development. We need not have a full understanding of the physics of solid-state electronics to be able to use a television; physicists do not need our direct help in continuing their work—just some money.

Medicine is different. Although it has more than its share of arcane complexity, it needs public cooperation to a much greater extent than other sciences. Without widespread cooperation, clinical trials would be impossible, as would the efficacious use of treatment strategies. For most chronic conditions a patient might meet with a physician for an hour or two a year, yet the treatment takes place continuously. For such cooperation the patient must understand the treatment and, in a deep sense, accept it; and of course, medical research needs money too. But how is this cooperation accomplished? For a long time it was through the power of authority[1], but in the modern world authority is no longer enough, if ever it was. Now the tactic most often taken is to provide the consuming public with illumination that explains the procedures, the theory and the evidence behind them, in the hopes of convincing the patient and the public to buy in.

The use of evidence in medical practice is emerging as a "new paradigm" to get the public's full cooperation. This audacious claim was made by the Evidence-Based Medicine Working Group in a 1992 article in the *Journal of the American*

Medical Association. The authors go on to explain that this new approach de-emphasizes intuition, unsystematic clinical experience and authority; they suggested supplanting them with rigorous use of formally gathered and analyzed empirical information. If only the emerging medical practice is evidence-based, what was medicine based on previously?

Obviously this claim is one of emphasis, reflecting a quantitative change, not a qualitative one. There is weak evidence that the empiricist school of medicine can be traced back to Acron of Akragas, a fifth century BC follower of Empedocles, the Sicilian philosopher and poet. Or perhaps medical empiricism began two hundred years later with Serapion of Alexandria. But there is no doubt that the clinical practices of Galen of Pergamum (ca.129–216) were firmly based on evidence. Galen was so prolific in recording his findings that if "publish or perish" were literally true, he would still be alive today. And, because of its quality, his work was enormously influential: so influential, that belief in his findings caused his followers to over-ride his methods. Let me illustrate this with the compelling example of the chambers of the uterus[2].

In Chapter 14 of his book, *On the Usefulness of the Parts,* Galen observed,

> Now though the neck (of the uterus) is single, Nature has not made just one hollow in the uteri. In the pig and certain other animals that must bear many fetuses, she has made many sinuses, but in man and animals resembling man, just as the whole body is double with right and left sides, so too there is one sinus placed on the right side of the uterus and another on the left.

He goes on to explain that the number of sinuses in the uterus matches the number of teats.

Despite ample opportunities to gather counter-evidence, including the spectacular anatomical drawings of Leonardo Da Vinci (1452–1509) (see Figure 1), this misconception of the character of the human uterus persisted for more than 1400 years. The anatomical studies of Andreas Vesalius (1514–1564) that correctly depict a single chambered human uterus, finally put this issue to rest, though not without apologies to Galen.

What took so long? We get a hint of an answer from the writings of Jacobus Sylvius of Amiens (1478–1555) who remarked that "any structure found in contemporary man that differed from the Galenical description could only be due to a later decadence and degeneration in mankind"—fourteen hundred years of supporting a conjecture that could be brought to question through the observation of a single dissection of a human female cadaver, and overthrown entirely when found repeatedly! We begin to get an understanding of the power of authority.

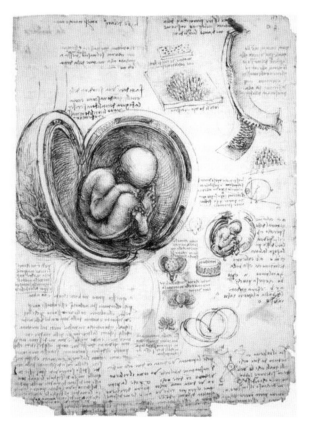

Figure 1 A page from Leonardo's *Notebooks*, "Studies of Embryos," ca. 1510–13, pen over red chalk. (Reproduced with permission from the Windsor Castle, Royal Library. ©Her Majesty Queen Elizabeth II.)

Of course the history of science is not this simple (Jaynes, 1966). We can begin with the Roman defilement of its Greek origins, as well as the oppressiveness thrown over science by the triumph of Augustine's ideas after the fall of Rome in 410; this signaled the dearth of anything original written in science until 9th century Basra. Then emerged the grand consilience of Arabic, Christian, Greek and Hebrew ideas that shone so brightly in Islamic Spain at the beginning of the second millennium. And finally, the Renaissance, in which the 16th century, which ushered in a thrilling crescendo of exploration and adventure, also practically invented the idea of nature, and with it, the beginning of modern biology.

But while the movement of Evidence-Based Medicine might date itself from 1991 or 1992, the common noun evidence-based medicine is surely much older.

A notable, and remarkably modern early example, is provided by the French physician Pierre Charles Alexandre Louis (1787–1872), who in <u>1835</u> published powerful empirical evidence[3] that bloodletting was not an effective treatment, thus overturning François Joseph Victor Broussais' (1772–1838) popular method of using leeches[4] to let blood.

In this book we will explore a number of examples of how looking at evidence can aid us in improving medical practice, and more particularly, how well-considered displays of carefully gathered data, in combination with thinking hard about what we see can provide great power in the search for illumination.

Chapter 1 is, in a very real sense, the middle of the story. It tells of two conflicting views of the public's right to know. On one side is a belief in the value of unadorned facts, on the other is the recognition that facts without understanding are more likely to lead to mischief than enlightenment. This conflict manifested itself in a 2010 law enacted in New York that requires the state's Health Department to make a map of cancer incidence available on-line along with plausible "causes" that can be overlain. Although both the Health Department and the American Cancer Society objected to the raw data being put "out there" with what they felt was insufficient explanation, the law's sponsor, Assemblyman Richard Brodsky, prevailed. In this chapter I illustrate why the concerns of experts should have been considered more carefully. This single example shows that we must concern ourselves with how to display information and also how to embed that display within a context that shrinks the likelihood of misunderstanding as much as possible.

The experience gained from the kerfuffle surrounding the broadcast of New York's cancer maps must be kept in the front of our vision as we next turn to how to communicate complex information correctly to a wide audience. A broad understanding of facts without including the often subtle and nuanced thinking required for their correct interpretation is not likely to yield a happy outcome. In Chapter 2 we drop back 70 years to introduce Will Burtin, a great graphic designer, who labored primarily in the medical field. Burtin's work provides us with a sample data set that illuminates the efficacy of what were then the newly emerging "wonder drugs" at fighting bacterial infections. We will use Burtin's data to show something of the breadth of display possibilities that now exist and how different kinds of displays can emphasize different aspects of the data's character. The greatest value of a good display is when it forces us to see what we never expected; in Chapter 3, we illustrate this and suggest that had these data been looked at more carefully in 1951, foreshadows of two different discoveries that took place in 1974 and 1985 respectively would have been apparent.

We shift gears next to focus more directly on using graphic displays to help illuminate the public's understanding. Chapters 4 and 5 both deal with US national reports on disease and suggest a number of ways that these reports could be improved so that their important topics could be more brightly illuminated.

Section II contains six chapters on how evidence combined with statistical thinking can help us understand and cope with some practical health decisions that most of us are likely to face. First we consider the areas of diabetes (Chapter 6), hip fractures (Chapter 7) and breast cancer (Chapter 8). Then we look afresh at some puzzles: in Chapter 9 we propose a way to project long-term effects from shorter-term data; in Chapter 10 we discuss the accuracy of psychiatric predictions of future criminal behavior, and we conclude this section (Chapter 11) with a careful look at the unique and remarkable success that Chinese medical researchers have had in duplicating Occidental medical breakthroughs.

Finally, in Section III, I conclude with a distressing puzzle. Repeatedly in history a better way is found and firmly established empirically. But remarkably it often does not catch on, or more specifically it does not catch on completely (remember Galen's two-horned uterus!). In Chapter 12 we look at the disappointing history of hand washing among physicians and reflect on what that might mean about the rapid adoption of checklists in emergency rooms. Peptic ulcers also make an appearance. Lastly, in Chapter 13, we take a wide view and note three other major improvements that were ignored.

SECTION I

Communicating with the Public

Introduction

For the healing sciences to achieve their full potential the public must participate. Assessing the efficacy of new treatments on lab animals can only advance us part of the way. To be able to make the leap from lab animals to humans requires clinical trials on humans. Sometimes such trials needs enormous numbers of participants.

One of the most famous examples of this was the 1954 Salk vaccine experiment (Francis, 1955). At that time polio was a serious threat to children, but even so it was relatively rare, about 50 per 100,000. In order to measure the efficacy of the Salk vaccine it needed to be tested on a sample that was large enough for the effect of the vaccine to manifest itself. About 200,000 children were randomly chosen to receive the vaccine and 57 were subsequently diagnosed with polio. The control group was about the same size but 142 contracted the disease (the rates per 100,000 were 28 and 71 respectively). The difference, 85 out of more than 400,000, was large enough for all to agree that it was extremely unlikely to have occurred by chance. This justified the vaccine's widespread use resulting in the essential eradication of polio in the industrialized world. A sample smaller than 400,000 would not have provided strong enough evidence.

The actual experiment was considerably more complex than what I have recounted, but this extract of the design is enough to make my point. For medical progress, hundreds of thousands of parents had to be convinced to allow their children to participate, knowing full well that the dependent variable of the experiment was the number of their children who contracted polio. Yet they agreed. They agreed because they were convinced of the importance of the result, and because not finding a solution was not an acceptable outcome.

The success of the Salk experiment has gone a long way toward making large-scale medical experiments acceptable. But the modern public requires evidence before it will put itself at risk in such experimentation. The public also requires evidence to justify the many billions of tax dollars spent on medical research in pursuit of similar miracles.

In the chapters of this section I will discuss modern attempts to communicate with the public. In all cases graphical methods were employed to convey what would have been too difficult to explain in prose.

Chapter 1 describes New York State's Health Department's attempt to comply with some over-zealous legislation regarding the communication of cancer incidence within the confines of the state. I try to explain some of the statistical subtleties behind why mapping raw data may be more dangerous than no data at all.

Chapter 2 begins in the 1930s in Nazi Germany as I tell the story of how Will Burtin, a modern master of graphical communication, emigrated to the United States to begin a remarkable career. We shall use one of his designs as a jumping-off point in a series of case studies to illuminate the efficacy of three "wonder drugs" in the treatment of bacterial infections. Of at least equal importance, it shows how there are many paths to salvation. Burtin's data then leads us, in Chapter 3, to a clever new display that, had it been constructed in 1951, would have provided a foreshadowing of scientific discoveries that lay decades in the future. It also provides a vivid reminder of how a graphic display is unique among scientific tools in forcing us to see what we never expected.

Chapter 4 examines the graphical methods used to communicate medical outcomes to the general public in a widely circulated federal report. I use this to illustrate how following some general rules for data display improves clarity and hence illumination.

And, finally, in Chapter 5 I argue for using just the right amount of creativity in developing health reports, neither too much nor too little. I feature the National Center for Health Statistics *Atlas of Mortality* as a shining example of public reporting done well. I also, alas, fall prey to the dark side in my snarky description of the Markle Foundation's foray into creativity run amok, the bizarre chartbook *Understanding USA*.

New York's cancer maps: What we don't know won't hurt us, it's what we do know that ain't

The legend of the Texas Sharpshooter

In the hill country of Texas stories are told of a legendary sharpshooter whose bullet-hole riddled barn bore the evidence of his expertise. On the barn was a crudely drawn target and in its centermost ring was a tight cluster of six bullet-holes. Over the target is written the inscription "Colt 45 at 100 yards." Admirers of the skill required for such a feat traveled from far and wide to visit the barn and pay homage to the memory of the marksman.

The sharpshooter's ex-wife, the only living witness to the feat, reports to anyone who would listen, that one day, during a drunken frenzy, her husband went outside and stood about 100 yards from the barn and spent the afternoon emptying box after box of ammunition in the general direction of his barn. When he sobered up the following morning, he went outside and surveyed the damage. He saw in the midst of the devastation that there was a cluster of six holes in the northwest corner of the barn. He ran inside and returned shortly with a brush and a can of white paint. He drew a target around the cluster and composed what was to become the famous inscription.

Of those who heard her, few understood. For many, their admiration only increased; for such marksmanship was difficult enough when sober—to have accomplished it while pie-eyed was remarkable indeed.

Facts without context are often likely to yield only misunderstanding of causal mechanisms.

1.1 Introduction: New York's cancer maps

On May 11, 2010 Danny Hakin of *The New York Times* reported that the web site of New York State's Health Department now contained an interactive cancer map in which the incidence of various kinds of cancer can be shown by Census block. In addition to showing cancer, the map also allows users to overlay it with potentially hazardous sites such as superfund sites, chemical storage locations and brown-fields[1]. Apparently the Health Department was forced to make these maps public when legislation sponsored by Assemblyman Richard Brodsky and State Senator Tom Libous was signed into law by Governor David A. Paterson, over the objections of the New York State Health Department and the American Cancer Society.

Assemblyman Brodsky defended the law, saying that this was the "first step in getting to answers about whether these (cancer) clusters are statistical accidents or related to an environmental cause." Claudia Hutton, director of public affairs for the Health Department said that they objected to making such data easily available because they were potentially misleading, that "an overlay of environmental-type facilities with new cancer cases might lead people to make incorrect conclusions . . . to be most useful to the public, health information needs to be provided with context."

Mr. Brodsky disagreed, saying "You bump against this question again and again: Should the government trust the people enough to tell them the truth?"

In a 2008 letter to the governor's office the American Cancer Society opposed the legislation, saying that "giving people potentially misleading information about the relative danger or safety of living or working in a specific neighborhood or region is no service to them."

Senator Libous dismissed such concerns proclaiming, "We believe that this is good, solid public health policy, that people should have this information."

Is this one of those policies that only makes sense if you say it fast? Let's take a slower look.

There are at least two principal concerns with making data like these broadly available to the lay public. The first is the ease that casual observers can make causal inferences. The second are the often subtle statistical effects that can make random fluctuations look real.

Causal inferences fall into one of two categories:

(i) Finding the cause of effects, and

(ii) Measuring the effects of causes.

1.2 John Snow's map of cholera: An early example

Finding the cause of effects is a task of insuperable difficulty. As an example let us reach back into mid-nineteenth century London when a cholera epidemic was killing many of the inhabitants of St. James Parish (Johnson, 2006). Dr. John Snow (1813–1858), a founding father of modern epidemiology, prepared his now famous map, which illustrated how he was able to trace the cause of the epidemic to drinking from the Broad Street pump (Figure 1.1). He removed its handle and, within days, the epidemic that had taken more than five hundred lives, sputtered to an end.

Does John Snow's success with this map support the case for making maps of unadjusted cancer data and some plausible causes public? Did it help Snow find the cause of the epidemic? What was the cause of the 1854 London epidemic? Was it the water drawn from the Broad Street pump? Or perhaps it was Frances Lewis' feces[2] that leaked out of a nearby cesspool? Frances Lewis was a five-month old child, who lived at 40 Broad Street and perished from cholera; she is widely considered to be the index case of that epidemic. Or was it the bacteria *Vibrio cholerae* in those feces? The Italian Filippo Pacini is now credited with being the first to identify this bacterium as the proximal cause of cholera in 1854, ironically the same year as the London epidemic. Is it really *V. cholerae*? Or is it the enterotoxin that it generates? You get the idea. As we learn more our judgment of what is the "true cause" keeps shifting. It is likely that at some time in the future research will reveal that it is some peculiar protein that interacts in an odd way to cause the disease. And even that is unlikely to be the end of it.

This is almost always the case when we try to find the cause of an effect. But measuring the effect of a cause is easier (although by no means easy). And, more important, once measured, it is eternal. Although what John Snow determined was the cause of the 1854 cholera epidemic has shifted over time, the effect of drinking from the Broad Street pump—the end of 570 lives—remains true.

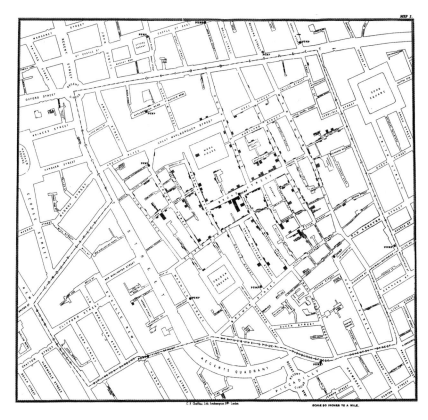

Figure 1.1 A map of the area near the Broad Street pump, taken from John Snow's 1855 book on the communication of cholera. The shaded bars indicate the number of deaths at that location. The pump is at the center of all of the deaths. Image courtesy of Wikimedia Commons.

Modern epistemology focuses on measuring the effects of causes[3]. It is deemed more fruitful to set aside questions like "does smoking cause cancer?" in favor of the quantitative question, "how much is your risk of cancer increased if you smoke?"

Superimposing plausible causes of various cancers over a map of incidence may yield some suggestive patterns, but the naïve drawing of causal inferences from such a display is almost surely likely to yield more mischief than illumination.

Yet counter-posed to this is John Snow's apparently successful use of this method. Is this possibility enough to justify New York's cancer maps? Before trying to answer this let us consider two things.

First, Snow did not simply draw his famous map and declare that the Broad Street pump was contaminated. The map just provided a neat summary of what was a pains-taking investigation. He went to the homes of the families of those who died, but were far from the pump to see if they had any connection. He found out about the Lewis family's waste disposal practices, and he investigated the drinking habits of brewery workers who worked near the pump but were under-represented among its victims. In short, the map might be considered a brilliant beginning of his investigation, but it was a long way from the end. How many of the users of New York's cancer maps are in a position to take such pains? Compare that with the number that might jump to an unwarranted, and ultimately unjustified, conclusion.

Second, there is strong evidence that his dramatic removal of the pump handle had little effect on the cholera epidemic. We suspect this because we now know how fragile and short-lived *V. cholerae* is outside of its host's body. Even without this knowledge, there was evidence in Snow's time that the epidemic had run its course. In Figure 1.2[4] we see the start of the epidemic with Francis Lewis' death on August 19. Then the disease grew slowly until August 31 when there was a huge increase in deaths, peaking the next day when more than 120

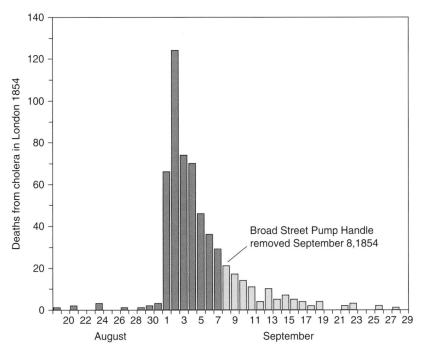

Figure 1.2 The daily number of deaths during the London cholera epidemic of 1854 showing that the epidemic had already begun to taper off well before the pump handle was removed on September 8th.

died. Then a decline began with the number of daily deaths shrinking steadily. The shading change in Figure 1.2 indicates the deaths after the pump handle was removed. But we see no dramatic shift; instead we see the tapering off that characterizes all epidemics as the number of potential victims diminishes. There is, alas, little evidence that Snow's action had any profound effect on the outcome of the course of the epidemic.

1.3 Finding the cause of the SAT score decline: *Post hoc ergo propter hoc*[5]

A more light-hearted example than cancer or cholera (and what isn't?) is shown in Figure 1.3a. In 1998 the College Board released 27 years of average scores on the SAT. Soon thereafter a fundamentalist group published a graph of those data augmented by a vertical line indicating the 1962 decision to ban prayer in public schools, obviously hinting at a causal connection (Figure 1.3b).[6]

As convincing as this evidence of the importance of prayer in the public schools might be, it still left the puzzle of why did the decline stop in the late 1970s and begin a slow and wobbly ascent? The Supreme Court did not reverse its school prayer decision. I may have found the answer, and indicated it through the inclusion of a second vertical line in 1977 marking both Elvis' death and the end of the SAT score decline. I also added the short note making explicit the causal message (Figure 1.3c) with a refrain from a popular Country and Western song.

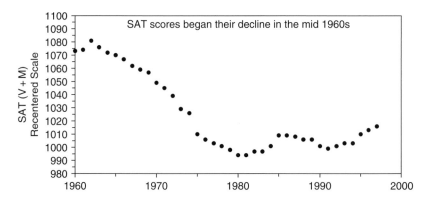

Figure 1.3a Average SAT scores for 27 years, showing a peak in 1962 that is followed by an 18-year decline.

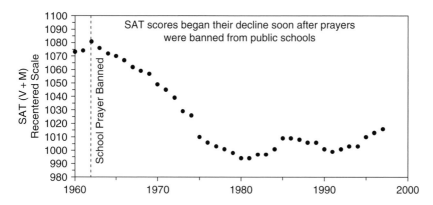

Figure 1.3b An augmentation of the SAT score plot indicating what some believe to be the proximal cause of the score decline.

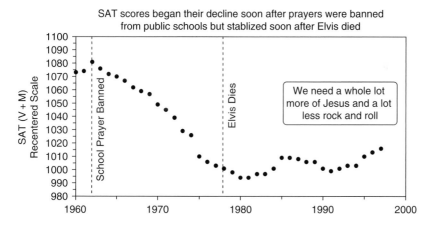

Figure 1.3c SAT scores began their decline soon after prayers were banned from public schools, but stabilized soon after Elvis died.

I would feel that this topic was not adequately discussed if I did not at least mention an alternative explanation for the SAT score decline, one that extensive research has given reasonable, though not conclusive, support. Specifically, that the score decline represented good news. In 1964 Lyndon Johnson's "War on Poverty" was beginning to gather momentum. One of the things that it did was provide additional support for higher education to help those on the economic margin. Those students tended to be on the education margin as well; their SAT scores were lower, on average, than those who had typically taken the test. Consequently, although the average SAT scores began to drop in 1964, the number of students who were considering college and hence opted to take the SAT increased dramatically. Supporting this interpretation was the decrease in SAT volume that accompanied decreases in educational funding during the Reagan administration in 1980.

I will not go further in the discussion of how New York's cancer maps can make the drawing of unsubstantiated causal claims too easy by letting the user overlay them with ancillary information. Next, let's look at a more subtle effect that manifests itself in these maps, as well as many others.

1.4 The danger of statistical ignorance

Let me illustrate how such maps can be misleading. Figure 1.4a is a map, closely akin to those of New York, of age adjusted kidney cancer rates. The counties shaded are those counties that are in the *lowest* 10% of the cancer distribution. We note that these healthy counties tend to be very rural, Midwestern, Southern and Western counties. So far, so good. It is both easy and tempting to make the inferential leap that this outcome is directly due to the clean living of the rural lifestyle—no air pollution, no water pollution, access to fresh food without additives, etc.

Figure 1.4b is another map of age adjusted kidney cancer rates. While it looks very much like Figure 1.4a, it differs in one important detail—the counties shaded are those counties that are in the *highest* 10% of the cancer distribution. Note that these ailing counties tend to be very rural, Midwestern, Southern and Western counties. If we hadn't already seen Figure 1.4a we would be tempted to infer that this outcome might be directly due to the poverty of the rural lifestyle—no access to good medical care, a high fat diet, and too much alcohol, too much tobacco.

If we were to plot Figure 1.4a on top of Figure 1.4b we would see that many of the shaded counties on one map are right next to the shaded counties in the other. What is going on?

What we are seeing is the effect of what is called "de Moivre's equation."[7] This equation provides a mathematical explanation of why small counties have much larger variation than large counties. A county with, say 100 inhabitants that has no cancer deaths would be in the lowest category of risk. But if it has one cancer death it would be among the highest. Counties like Manhattan or Los Angeles or Miami/Dade with millions of inhabitants do not bounce around like that. Hence on all variables measured we should always expect to find small counties at both extremes.

If we plot the age-adjusted[8] cancer rates against county population this result becomes clearer still (Figure 1.5). We see the typical triangular shape in which

Lowest kidney cancer death rates

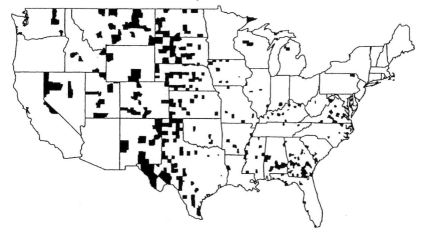

Figure 1.4a The counties of the United States with the lowest 10% age-standardized death rates for cancer of kidney/urethra for US males, 1980–1989 (from Gelman & Nolan, 2002, p. 15), reprinted with permission.

Highest kidney cancer death rates

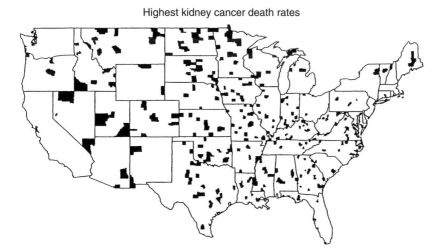

Figure 1.4b The counties of the United States with the highest 10% age-standardized death rates for cancer of kidney/urethra for US males, 1980–1989 (from Gelman & Nolan, 2002, p. 14), reprinted with permission.

when the population is small (left side of the graph) there is wide variation in cancer rates, from 20 per hundred thousand to zero. When county populations are large (right side of the graph) there is very little variation with all counties at about five cases per hundred thousand of population.

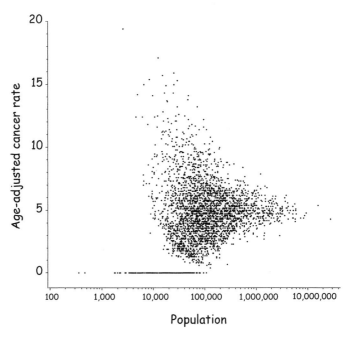

Figure 1.5 Age adjusted kidney cancer rates for all US counties in 1980–1989 shown as a function of the log of the county population.

This is a compelling example of how someone who looked only at, say, Figure 1.4a, and not knowing about de Moivre's equation might draw incorrect inferences and give incorrect advice (e.g. if you are at risk of kidney cancer you should move to the wide open spaces of rural America).

We see exactly this effect in some New York State county maps (the effect is magnified with maps of smaller entities, like zip-codes or Census tracts). For example, in tiny Essex County (county 20 in the extreme north-east), which lies mostly within the Adirondack Park, there appears to be an extremely excessive incidence of non-Hodgkin's lymphoma among women (Figure 1.6a), but for men it is just as far *below* average (Figure 1.6b).

Current understanding of this disease does not suggest that there should be large differences between its relative incidence in men and women. In populous counties (e.g. Kings, Queens, Nassau) there is no difference between the sexes.

I suspect that it was concerns like these that were expressed by the professionals at the Cancer Society and the Health Department that went unheeded by Assemblyman Brodsky and Senator Libous when they insisted that unadjusted data for small areas be made available to the unsuspecting people of New York.

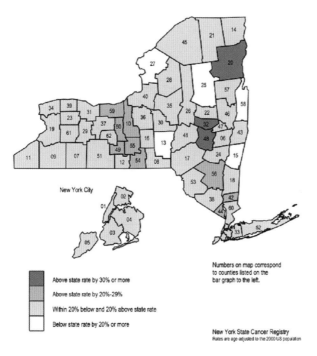

Non-Hodgkin Lymphoma
Age-Adjusted Incidence Rates among Females
New York State, by County, 2003-2007

Above state rate by 30% or more

Above state rate by 20%-29%

Within 20% below and 20% above state rate

Below state rate by 20% or more

Numbers on map correspond
to counties listed on the
bar graph to the left.

New York State Cancer Registry
Rates are age-adjusted to the 2000 US population

Figure 1.6a Non-Hodgkin's lymphoma among females. Note the high rate in Essex County (county 20 in the north-east).

It is said that there are two kinds of lawyers: one tells you that you can't do it, and the other tells you how to do it. The decision of which one to hire is easy. I fear that I have come across as the wrong kind of lawyer, for I have taken great care to show how the naked empiricism that has us looking at cancer incidence data on a geographic background, combined with an overlay of plausible causal factors might do more damage than the re-establishment of the inquisition. That is not the message I want to leave you with. Massive data gathering and modern display and analysis technology are important tools that, when used wisely and with knowledge, can be mighty allies in the search for solutions to difficult problems. But such powerful tools should be kept out of the hands of children and adults who don't understand their stringent limitations.

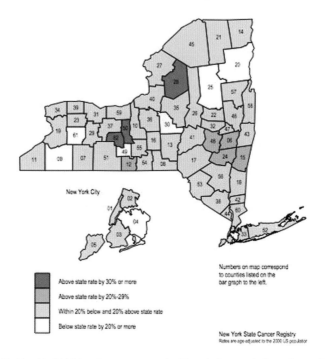

Non-Hodgkin Lymphoma
Age-Adjusted Incidence Rates among Males
New York State, by County, 2003-2007

Numbers on map correspond
to counties listed on the
bar graph to the left.

Above state rate by 30% or more

Above state rate by 20%-29%

Within 20% below and 20% above state rate

Below state rate by 20% or more

New York State Cancer Registry
Rates are age-adjusted to the 2000 US population

Figure 1.6b Non-Hodgkin's lymphoma among males. Note the low rate in Essex County (county 20 in the north-east). http://www.nyhealth.gov/statistics/cancer/registry/cntymaps/.

Let me conclude with the Will Rogers' wise observation that formed the title of this chapter,

"What we don't know won't hurt us, it's what we do know that ain't."

I fear that with such information more widely available than the knowledge to use them wisely it can be too easy for incorrect causal inferences to be drawn and thence communities to be unfairly stigmatized.

This concern brings us to the principal theme of this book, our great need for illumination. Without such illumination the spirit of the Texas Sharpshooter, his very bones now long dust, will continue to haunt us.

CHAPTER 2

A centenary celebration for Will Burtin: A pioneer of scientific visualization

2.1 Introduction to Will Burtin

The next chapter of our story begins in Nazi Germany. It's the summer of 1938 and Europe stands on the brink of war. A year earlier, Josef Goebbels, the Reich Minister of Propaganda, had asked 29 year old Wilhelm Burtin[1] to become Propaganda Director at the Ministry (Semmelweis & Codell, 1983). The brilliant young designer played for time. On the surface this seemed like a remarkable opportunity, but Burtin's wife Hilde Munk was Jewish. Although Kristalnacht still lay almost a year in the future, it did not take a seer to foresee the problems that Jews would encounter in the 3rd Reich. So Hilde wrote to her American cousin, Max Munk, and asked if he would sponsor their immigration to the US. But the clock was ticking and it wasn't prudent to stall Goebbel's advances too long. Then Adolf Hitler, the Fuhrer himself, repeated Goebbel's offer and Burtin could stall no longer. Happily, at this moment Max's sponsorship came through and in the summer of 1938 the couple left for America and Wilhelm became Will Burtin (Figure 2.1).

Despite his limited English[2] he was an almost instantaneous success. Within months of his arrival he won a contract to design the Federal Works Agency Exhibition for the US Pavilion at the New York World's Fair. By 1939 he had designed the cover for the World's Fair issue of *The Architectural Forum*

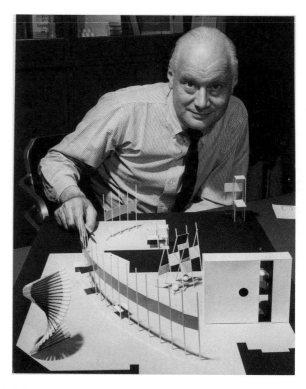

Figure 2.1 Will Burtin in a detail of an image produced by the Upjohn Company, photograph by the Mechanical Development department for the *Visual Communications 1957* exhibit. Copyright © Pfizer Inc. Reproduced with Permission.

magazine, which won the Art Directors' Club medal for cover design. Thus began a rich career, which included a long relationship with Upjohn Pharmaceuticals. During this time he was responsible for the design of much of the content of Upjohn's magazine *Scope*, which was focused on communicating technical material to physicians. A 1951 example of one of his designs from *Scope* forms the basis of Section 2.3 of this chapter.

2.2 The cell

The 1950s were a transformational time in biology and, more specifically, 1953 was *annus mirabilis*. In this one remarkable year Watson and Crick published their famous paper on the double helix structure of DNA. In the same issue of *Nature* Wilkins, Stokes & Wilson published a paper providing the X-ray

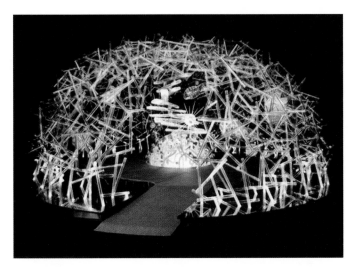

Figure 2.2 Photograph. Cell (24 ft) exhibit exterior, 1958. Copyright © Pfizer Inc. Reproduced with Permission.

crystallographic evidence to support Watson & Crick, and in that same issue Rosalind Franklin and Ray Gosling added further support and suggested that the phosphate backbone of the DNA molecule lies on the outside of the structure. A week later Watson & Crick added detailed speculation on how the base pairing in the double helix allows DNA to replicate. Information about detailed cellular structure poured from the literature, but because it was hard to visualize it was hard to integrate. Burtin convinced Upjohn president Jack Gauntlett that it would be worthwhile to fund the construction of a giant (24 feet across and 12 feet high) model of a human red blood cell that would provide all the details thus far known about it. It contained structures seen in electron microscopes but not yet explained and embodied modern scientific visualization on a grand scale. Burtin's cell (Figure 2.2) was unveiled in San Francisco at the 1958 meeting of the American Medical Association. It was the star of the convention and subsequently traveled widely.

2.3 The impact of three antibiotics on a variety of bacteria

In the post World War II world antibiotics were called "wonder drugs" for they provided quick and easy cures for what had previously been intractable diseases. Data were being gathered to aid in learning which drug worked best for what bacterial infection. Being able to see the structure of drug performance was an enormous aid for practitioners and scientists alike. In the Fall of 1951 Burtin published a graph showing the performance of the three most popular antibiotics on 16 different bacteria. The data that were used in his display are shown in Table 2.1. The entries of the table are the concentrations (in milligrams/deciliter—mg/dl) of the antibiotic required to halt the growth of the bacteria in vitro. The variable "Gram staining" describes the reaction of the bacteria to this stain. The stain is named after its inventor Hans Christian Gram (1853–1938), who developed the technique in 1884 to discriminate between two types of bacteria with similar clinical symptoms: *Streptococcus pneumoniae* and *Klebsiella pneumoniae*. Gram-positive bacteria are those that are stained dark blue or violet; Gram-negative bacteria do not react that way.

TABLE 2.1

Bacteria	Antibiotic			Gram staining
	Penicillin	Streptomycin	Neomycin	
Aerobacter aerogenes	870	1	1.6	negative
Bacillus anthracis	0.001	0.01	0.007	positive
Brucella abortus	1	2	0.02	negative
Diplococcus pneumoniae	0.005	11	10	positive
Escherichia coli	100	0.4	0.1	negative
Klebsiella pneumoniae	850	1.2	1	negative
Mycobacterium tuberculosis	800	5	2	negative
Proteus vulgaris	3	0.1	0.1	negative
Pseudomonas aeruginosa	850	2	0.4	negative
Salmonella (Eberthella) typhosa	1	0.4	0.008	negative
Salmonella schottmuelleri	10	0.8	0.09	negative
Staphylococcus albus	0.007	0.1	0.001	positive
Staphylococcus aureus	0.03	0.03	0.001	positive
Streptococcus faecalis	1	1	0.1	positive
Streptococcus hemolyticus	0.001	14	10	positive
Streptococcus viridans	0.005	10	40	positive

Burtin, who to my knowledge, had no training as a statistician, nevertheless made a variety of wise choices in the display of these data that he constructed (Figure 2.3).

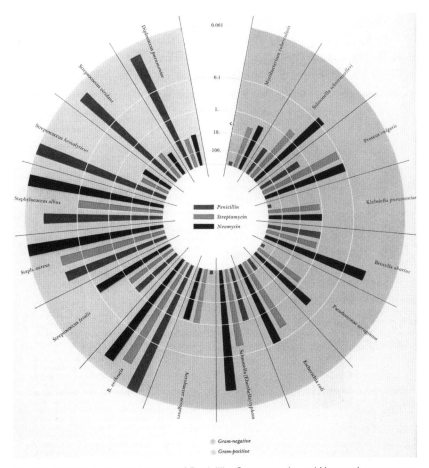

Burtin's diagram compares impacts of Penicillin, Streptomycin and Neomycin on a range of bacteria (*Scope*, Fall 1951). Copyright © Pfizer Inc. Reproduced with Permission.

Figure 2.3 Will Burtin's graphic depiction of the data from Table 2.1.
Antibacterial ranges of Neomycin, Penicillin and Streptomycin: The chart compares the in vitro sensitivities to Neomycin of some of the common pathogens (Gram-positive in red and Gram-negative in blue) with their sensitivities to Penicillin and Streptomycin. The effectiveness of the antibiotics is expressed as the highest dilution in μg/ml, which inhibits the test organism. High concentrations are inward from the periphery; consequently the length of the colored bar is proportional to the effectiveness.

His display is a direct lineal descendent of Florence Nightingale's famous Rose, in which the radii of the segments convey the amount of the data, rather than a traditional pie chart in which the angle of each segment is the carrier of the information. Burtin does several clever things in this display, two of them, of special interest, are described here.

First, he saw the huge range of values that the data took and realized that some sort of re-expression was necessary. He chose a logarithmic transformation. Such a re-expression is obvious to someone with statistical training, but it is reassuring that a designer should come to the same conclusion. The box plots in Figure 2.4a show the distributions of performance for each drug after log transformation, oriented so that better performance is at the top.

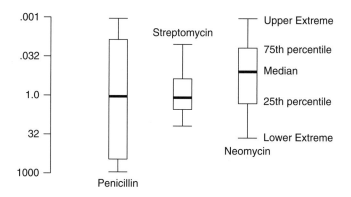

Figure 2.4a Three box plots showing the distributions of response that the 16 bacteria had to each of the antibiotics. Their symmetry indicates that the log transformation worked properly.

We see immediately that the transformation has worked in that the resulting distributions are symmetric without having unduly long tails. In addition, we can see that there is a far greater variation in the performance of Penicillin than in the other two drugs. Why? A dot plot that identifies Gram-positive and Gram-negative bacteria shows that Penicillin works far better for Gram-positive bacteria than for Gram-negative, a differential performance that is not evident for the other two drugs.

Burtin obviously noticed this and so he visually segregated the bacteria that were Gram-positive from those that were Gram-negative.

His resulting display is compact, accurate and informative. But with the wisdom borne of a half century of work on statistical display and exploratory data analysis, can we improve matters? An obvious nit is his omission of a circular reference line at .01. When interpolating between reference points humans have a tough time with a log scale. Thus it seems useful to provide as many intermediate way-points as possible so that linear interpolation is not too far off. But,

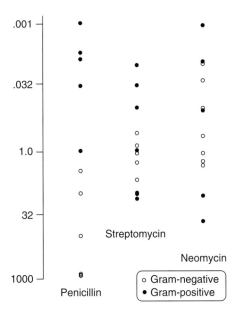

Figure 2.4b A dot plot of the same data as in Figure 2.4a showing that the greater variability observed for Penicillin was because of Penicillin's greater divergent efficacy for Gram-positive vs. Gram-negative bacteria.

perhaps it isn't important to judge accurately between 0.1 and 0.001. If so, this level of visual precision might be sufficient.

A place where real improvement may be possible is in the ordering of the bacteria. Let us consider just the Gram-positive bacteria; suppose we order the graph by the success rate of Penicillin, one possible display is shown in Figure 2.5.

Now we can see clearly that for Gram-positive bacteria, except *Streptococcus faecalis*, Penicillin works well, although for Staph infections Neomycin seems to have an edge. The peculiar behavior of *Streptococcus faecalis* will form one of the two supports of the theme of Chapter 3.

The second panel of this display, Figure 2.5b, would then be the Gram-negative bacteria, this time ordered by the effectiveness of Neomycin.

From even a cursory examination of this two-panel display we can easily decide which drug is best for what bacteria. We note that, for these bacteria at least, Streptomycin is dominated by the other two drugs. I contend that this two-panel display, although it lacks the compactness of Burtin's original design, has a small edge in exposing the underlying structure of drug effectiveness. I suspect that the rank order of the bacteria in each panel exposes an underlying

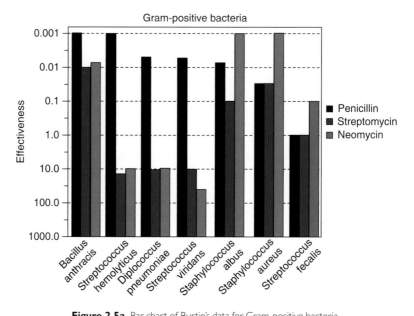

Figure 2.5a Bar chart of Burtin's data for Gram-positive bacteria.

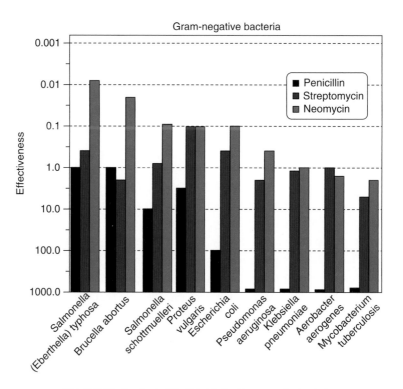

Figure 2.5b Bar chart of Burtin's data for Gram-negative bacteria.

molecular structure, but I leave it to others to uncover its meaning. In the next section we will look at a large number of alternative displays.

2.4 Going beyond Burtin—on the many paths to understanding

It has been more than two centuries since the formal invention of statistical graphics, and in that time they have become a mainstay in modern life. One cannot open a newspaper or magazine, or turn on a TV newscast without being confronted by them. And so it is not surprising that we have become pretty good at both reading and constructing them, although just how good was something of a surprise.

As part of the centenary celebration of Will Burtin's birth a contest was proposed to the readers of the statistical magazine *Chance*. The challenge was to construct a display of Burtin's 1951 data. Sixty-five readers of *Chance* worldwide responded. For the most part the results are very impressive indeed. In this section I will present a subset of the submissions. I chose these particular displays for two reasons. First, obviously, because they provided a clear view of one or more aspects of the data, and second, because they show how diverse are the graphical tools now available. The quality and diversity astonished me.

2.5 Purpose

Any design must begin with a statement of purpose. There are four purposes of graphs:

1 Exploration—a private discussion between the data and the graph maker about the character of the data. When this is the primary purpose the greatest value of the display is when it forces the viewer to see what he or she never expected.

2 Communication—a discussion between the graph maker and other people about the aspects of the data that the graph maker feels are most critical for the issue at hand.

3 Calculation—a nomograph, in which the graphic performs some calculation to allow the user to see a result without doing the arithmetic.

4 Decoration—the graph is used as a visual element of a presentation to attract the viewer's attention.

Although graphs often must serve multiple purposes, the optimal display for one purpose is usually not the same as for others, and so some hierarchy of purpose must be made. This is the first decision that must be made by the graph maker. For the Burtin data we expect that the displays would have communication as their primary goal, which presupposes that the graph maker has privately done some serious exploration to learn what messages are there to be communicated.

2.6 Questions to be answered

The second step is to decide what are the key questions that the data were gathered to answer. For these data the primary questions must surely be:

(i) What bacteria does this drug kill?

(ii) What drug kills this bacterium?

(iii) Does the descriptive variable "gram staining" help us make decisions?

(iv) How do the bacteria group vis-à-vis their reaction to the antibiotics?

(v) How do the antibiotics group with respect to their efficacy in controlling the bacteria?

At first blush one would think that (ii) is the key clinical question. For it would naturally result when a patient presents with a particular kind of infection, and the physician would want to know what is the most efficacious treatment. But, in 1951, when antibiotics were still new, question (i) might have assumed greater significance. A good display will answer one of these, a great display will answer both, while at the same time providing a clear overall picture of the battles between these bacteria and these antibiotics. Question (iii) is closely allied to both (ii) and (iv). If we cannot identify the specific bacterium, we can still know how it reacts to Gram stain. That may provide help in choosing an antibiotic. Question (v) is a deeper scientific question, for the grouping of the bacteria with respect to their reaction to antibiotics can provide taxonomic information.

2.7 Memorable

A great display should be memorable in that you should take away from it an overall picture of what is going on that is more than merely the details which were available from the original data matrix. To accomplish this the display needs to convey *coherence*, a unity of perception that is greater than just the sum of its parts. The best example of this is Minard's famous plot of Napoleon's failed Russian campaign (Figure 2.6) in which the river of the French army streams across the Russian steppes in the warmth of the summer of 1812 and trickles

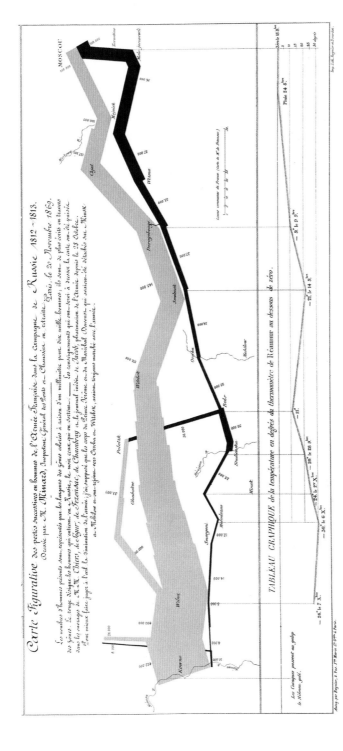

Figure 2.6 Charles Joseph Minard's 1869 plot of Napoleon's ill-fated Russian campaign. The width of the metaphorical river represents the size of Napoleon's army; its location represents the location of the army; its color tells us the direction of travel. The line at the bottom shows the temperature.

back across the Polish border in the midst of the terrible winter. The memory of the graph transcends the series of data points from which it was constituted.

To answer these questions requires thoughtful analyses and careful decisions about the scale of the graph, the visual metaphor that is used to represent the data, and the order in which the data are presented. In the following we shall see how some of the most talented graph makers in the world chose to address the problem. My annotations indicate the choices that were made and what might have been tried to improve them.

2.8 The dog on the night of the murder[3]

Before discussing any of these displays explicitly it is sensible to mention what was to me one of the most remarkable characteristic of all but two of the submissions; they were all in a log scale. Of course, when we see that the values of the minimum inhibitory concentrations (MICs) covered a range of about a million to one, any statistician would immediately transform. So it is easy to lose sight of how rare is this insight in the general population. When I tried this same exercise on undergraduates in an introductory statistics course the proportion who used a transformation was vanishingly small. So my applause to all entrants (save two) who did the transformation *pro forma*.

2.9 Fifteen displays about one thing

Entry 1—A remarkable display aimed at communication, exploration and decoration

In this display the three antibiotics are represented by three vertical lines and the various bacteria as connecting lines whose character indicated their Gram staining response. Of course the scale chosen was logarithmic and the various bacteria were shown delightfully by their micro-photographs. The location of crossing of the antibiotic axes by the bacterial lines shows the antibiotics' efficacy. The grouping of the lines shows their similarity of reaction (much more on this in Chapter 3). If this display has a shortcoming it stems from its impressive ambition. It is hard to discern which bacterium is which as the lines that connect performance with identifier get visually jumbled. But it is a wonderful beginning for this exhibition.

Entry 2—Summarizing results indelibly

In this display the data are averaged over all bacteria within each of the Gram staining categories and the average amount is shown in pill form. For

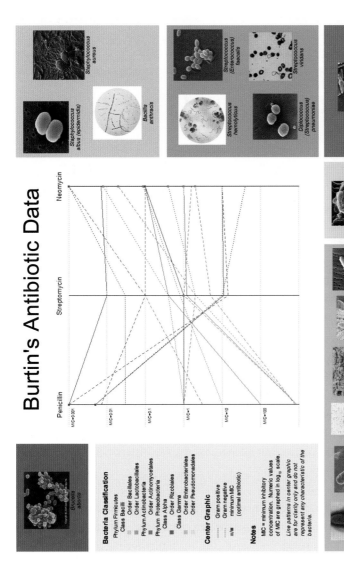

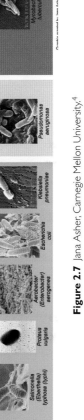

Figure 2.7 Jana Asher, Carnegie Mellon University.[4]

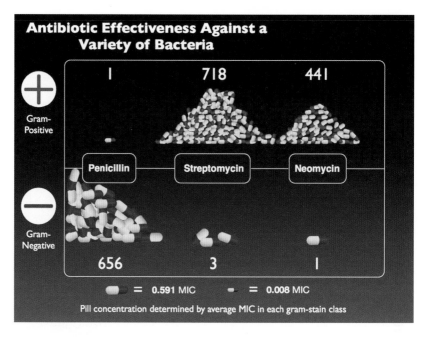

Figure 2.8 Troy Brandt, Stanford University.

Gram-positive bacteria Penicillin is the clear winner, and it is hard to forget the pile of 718 pills of Streptomycin that would be required to do the job. In parallel we can easily see that with Gram-negative bacteria Neomycin is the antibiotic of choice. It is important to note that the red pills are 74 times larger than the blue ones, and so even if only one red pill of Neomycin is required for a Gram-negative bacteria, it is a whopping big one!

The display does not allow us to look at the performance against any specific bacterium within the larger Gram class, but the picture we obtain is clear and unforgettable. A decorative, but memorable, display with punch.

Entry 3—A decorative hybrid display joining a table with drops of antibiotics

This display circumvents the need to use a log transformation of the MICs by using a visual transformation. It uses the perceived volume of the droplet to represent the MIC and manages to convey the qualitative feeling of the differences in effective dosages. It does this because we perceive the diameter of the drop which is proportional to the cube root of the volume. The cube-root transformation goes a long way toward taming the great variations in MICs.

In addition it is a hybrid display in that it also reproduces the data table. In fact, one might think of this display as a table augmented with some graphic

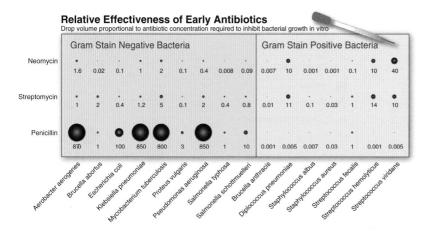

Relative Effectiveness of Early Antibiotics

Drop volume proportional to antibiotic concentration required to inhibit bacterial growth in vitro

	Gram Stain Negative Bacteria									Gram Stain Positive Bacteria						
Neomycin	1.6	0.02	0.1	1	2	0.1	0.4	0.008	0.09	0.007	10	0.001	0.001	0.1	10	40
Streptomycin	1	2	0.4	1.2	5	0.1	2	0.4	0.8	0.01	11	0.1	0.03	1	14	10
Penicillin	870	1	100	850	800	3	850	1	10	0.001	0.005	0.007	0.03	1	0.001	0.005

Aerobacter aerogenes · Brucella abortus · Escherichia coli · Klebsiella pneumoniae · Mycobacterium tuberculosis · Proteus vulgaris · Pseudomonas aeruginosa · Salmonella typhosa · Salmonella schottmuelleri · Brucella anthracis · Diplococcus pneumoniae · Staphylococcus albus · Staphylococcus aureus · Streptococcus fecalis · Streptococcus hemolyticus · Streptococcus viridans

Figure 2.9 Benjamin Lauderdale, Princeton; Katherine Lauderdale, Harvard.

elements. It forcefully tells us that if the bacterium is Gram positive use Penicillin (except for two of the Streptococci and the Diplococcus), and if it is Gram negative use Neomycin.

It might have done a somewhat better job if the bacteria were ordered by something other than the alphabet, but that is only a nit. It forms a compelling memory of the variation in dosage that exists, and helps a clinician formulate an evidence-based treatment protocol.

Entry 4. An unsuccessful attempt to escape Flatland using an enhanced scatterplot

The goal of this display is to think of the three antibiotics as the axes in a three-dimensional space. But faced with the limitations of plotting on a plane the graph maker opted to project the data onto the plane formed by just two antibiotics. Thus in this display each bacterium's response to Neomycin is plotted against that for Streptomycin in a scatter plot on a log scale oriented so that more effective is to the right/top. A fine idea, but it doesn't scale up to more than two drugs very well. Instead of a third dimension, Penicillin's effectiveness is shown by the size of the plotting point (bigger is better) and Gram staining is shown by the plotting point's color. This design's strength is that it shows the strong linear relationship between the effectiveness of Neomycin and Streptomycin directly, and the fact that Neomycin is better for almost all bacteria, but it is hard to see very much about Penicillin's relative performance.

As we will see in Chapter 3, this same approach but with Penicillin substituting for Streptomycin, would have been especially revealing.

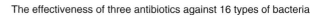

The effectiveness of three antibiotics against 16 types of bacteria

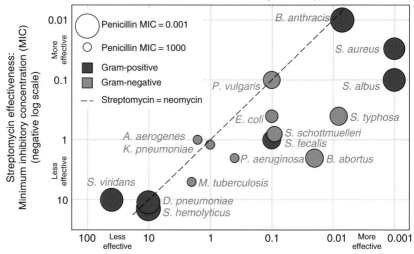

Figure 2.10 Lawrence B. Finer and Christian C. Ryan, New York, NY.

Entry 5—Pseudo 3-D, another unsuccessful attempt to escape Flatland

Effectiveness of 3 antibiotics on 16 bacteria

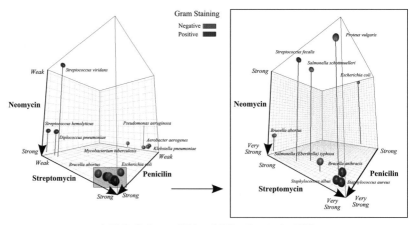

Antibiotic effectiveness as Minimum Inhibitory Concentrations (MIC).

Figure 2.11 Pierre Dangauthier, London, UK.

This display uses a pseudo 3-D display without any transformation of the data. To show fine structure it uses an inset (the right panel). It cannot scale up to more than three drugs. It is clumsy at answering some questions and the resulting picture is far from a memorable image.

Entry 6—Bars

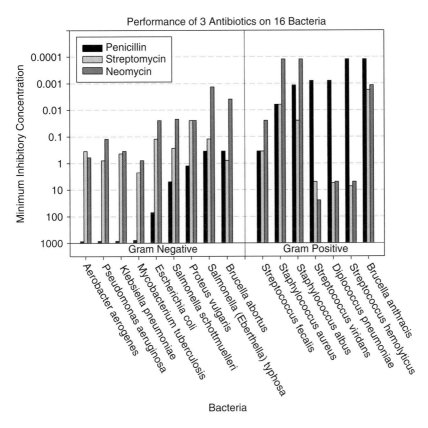

Figure 2.12a Donald Schopflocher, University of Alberta.

This display does a good job of presenting a coherent picture of the data. The log scale allows us to make distinctions among the various efficacies, Gram-positive and Gram-negative bacteria are visually separated, and the metaphor "bigger = better" is employed. The bacteria are ordered by the efficacy of Penicillin. I have reasons for great affection for this design, not the least of which is because it was the same one I came up with initially. But with the wisdom borne of seeing many other alternatives, my ardor has cooled somewhat. However,

Effectiveness of three antibiotics against a variety of bacteria.

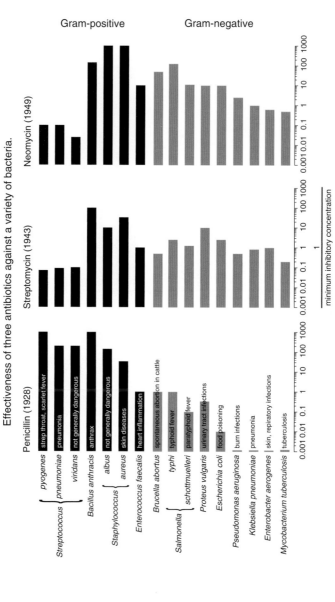

Figure 2.12b Justin Talbot, Stanford University.

before we move on to other alternatives it is worthwhile to note that one could easily augment this design with additional information (see Figure 2.12b) and thus convey more than just the response of bacteria to antibiotics, but also a greater depth of understanding about the diseases those bacteria cause.

Such augmentation is not unique to a bar chart design; indeed it could be added to most designs. The lesson to be learned is that the less space that is used up by non-data figurations ("Chart Junk" in Edward Tufte's evocative phrase) the more space is available for additional information; which segues us neatly to the next design.

Entry 7—Dots

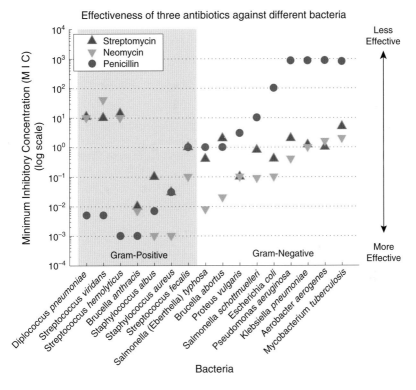

Figure 2.13 Mindy Chang, Stanford University.

The bar chart is a clean and simple display, but the bars are redundant and serve only to hold up the top line of the bar, which carries all of the information. Thus efficiency is well served by emphasizing the top and eliminating the bar. One such plot is shown as Figure 2.13. The Gram staining was visually separated, the dots representing a particular antibiotic were color coded, and the bacteria were ordered (approximately) by the efficacy of Penicillin. Thus we can compare bacteria and we can compare drugs. It has two shortcomings. First, to decode the display you must first memorize the legend, so that you know that a blue circle is Penicillin, etc. This means that you must "read" the display, rather than just "see" it. The second difficulty is that a collection of dots rarely provides a memorable image.

Entry 8—A more evocative plotting symbol

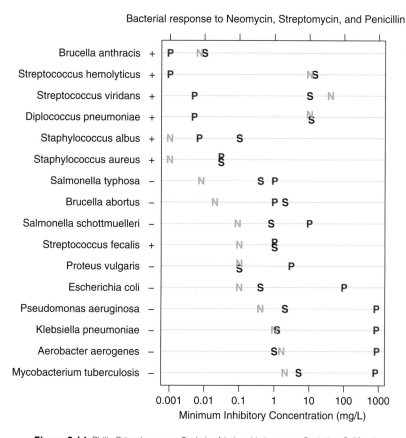

Bacterial response to Neomycin, Streptomycin, and Penicillin

Figure 2.14 Philip Price, Lawrence Berkeley National Laboratory, Berkeley, California.

The dot plot of Figure 2.14 is similar in many ways to that shown in Figure 2.13, except that instead of using three different geometric shaped dots as the plotting symbols to represent the three antibiotics, it uses the three letters P, S and N, thus obviating the need for a legend. This version can now be seen and legend memorization is no longer required. This also drastically reduces the likelihood of error. This same strategy should be used whenever possible on other graphical formats—for example we should label lines on a plot directly and not through a legend. How the bacteria in this version are ordered is not immediately obvious, although it is surely related to the bacteria's overall drug resistance. Last, a closer look suggests that there is something funny about *Streptococcus faecalis*. But this display is still just a bunch of dots; there is no coherent picture.

Entry 9—Connecting the dots

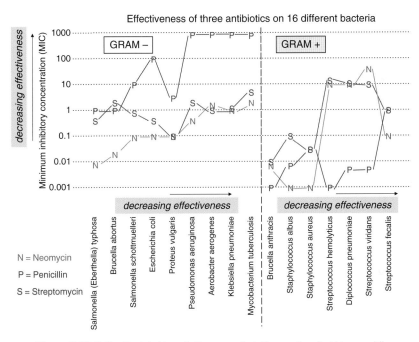

Figure 2.15 Céline Dartois, Novartis Pharmaceuticals Corporation, East Hanover, NJ.

One way to transform a disjointed plot filled with dots into a more unified picture, is to connect the dots that go together. Some might complain that doing so creates a false impression, for the axis listing the bacteria has no real metric. Well, phooey! All that heeding such a complaint will get you is to miss what you might have found. In Figure 2.15 the dots are connected after arranging the bacteria in order of increasing resistance to the drugs, after stratifying by Gram stain reaction.

Entry 10—Adding words

I gotta use words when I talk to you

    T.S. Eliot in *Sweeney Agonistes*

There are two kinds of good displays:

A *strongly good display* is one that tells you everything you want to know just by looking at it, and

A *weakly good display* is one that tells you everything you want to know just by looking at it, once you know what to look for.

We can transform a weakly good display into a strongly good one by adding explanatory labels. Figure 2.16 does precisely this. In case you were not able to figure out what was going on this display tells you in both words and picture. After seeing it there is no further excuse for ignorance about what antibiotic is effective against which bacteria. It also shows how to put the space saved by eliding the bars (in Figure 2.12) to good use. Getting rid of non-data figurations leaves room for more information, or in this case, for interpretive prose.

Entry 11—Small Multiples: I

Trying to display three or more dimensional data on a two-dimensional plane is always a tough assignment. There are many schemes that have been tried—Figure 2.11 is a common approach. Another possibility is to use a single small icon to represent the multidimensional structure. In Figure 2.17 the icon used to represent each bacterium is a triangle in which the distance of each vertex from the center was proportional to the log of the amount of antibiotic needed; the larger the icon the more resistant the bacterium. Icons of similar shape represent bacteria of similar patterns of resistance. Although this kind of display may have promise, to do better would require that the placement of the icons onto the two-dimensional plane be done more thoughtfully.

Entry 12—Small Multiples: II

The display shown in Figure 2.18 uses a different icon to represent each bacterium, one that is more easily decoded. It also arranges the icons in a way that allows us to answer questions about bacteria resistance easily. Looking within an icon provides easy identification of the best drug for a particular bacterium.

The horizontal line represents the maximum practical dosage (who can forget the piles of pills necessary shown in Figure 2.8) and so effective treatment is represented by the bars that go downward. It tells us that for some bacteria effective treatments are not yet in hand.

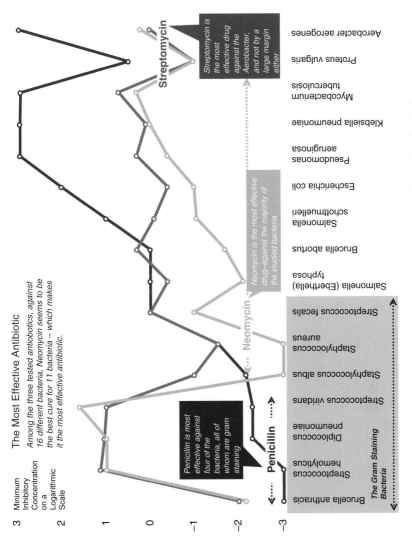

Figure 2.16 Dibyojyoti Haldar, Fast Moving Consumer Goods, Bangalore, India.

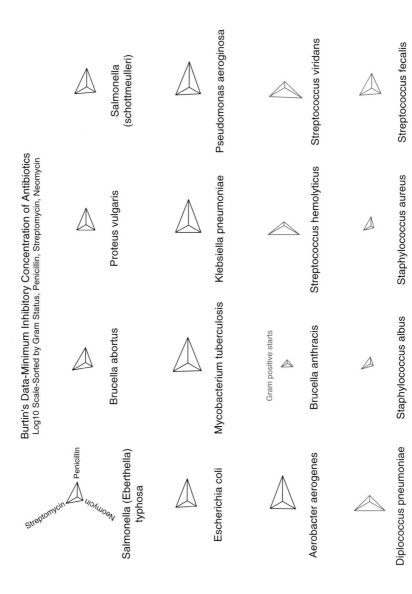

Figure 2.17 Georgette Asherman, Direct Effect LLC, Fort Lee, NJ.

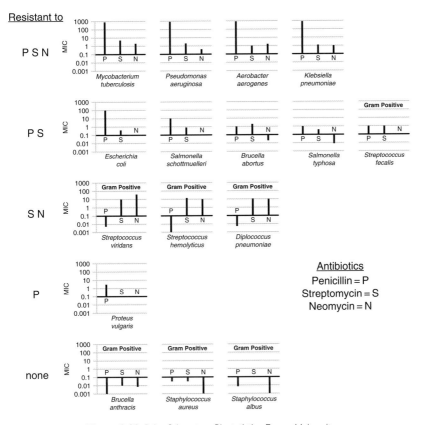

Figure 2.18 Brian Schmotzer, Biostatistics, Emory University.

The third row of this display should draw attention. All three bacteria have essentially the same profile of response to the three antibiotics. Two of them are Streptococci and one is Diplococcus. Why is that? A discussion of this observation forms the core of Chapter 3 and so I will defer further discussion until then.

Entry 13—Polygons

This display uses elements from Figures 2.17 and 2.18. Like Figure 2.17 it uses a polygon icon to represent the efficacy of the antibiotics, however in this case the each vertex is a bacterium. Like Figure 2.17 it represents the efficacy of the antibiotic with a point on the radius from the center of the polygon to its vertex; the metaphor is smaller equals more effective. Like Figure 2.18 it organizes the location of each bacterium wisely. It orders the bacteria around the icon carefully so that the polygon thus formed is smooth. The two panels of the display represent the two Gram stain conditions. Note that at a glance we see for the

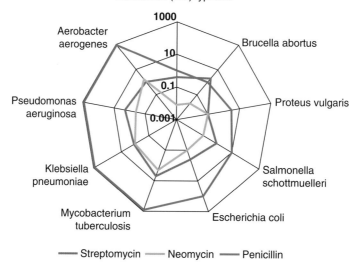

Negative Gram Staining

Salmonella (Ebt) typhosa

1000

Aerobacter aerogenes

10

Brucella abortus

0.1

Pseudomonas aeruginosa

0.001

Proteus vulgaris

Klebsiella pneumoniae

Salmonella schottmuelleri

Mycobacterium tuberculosis

Escherichia coli

—— Streptomycin —— Neomycin —— Penicillin

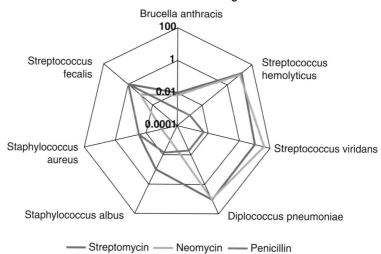

Positive Gram Staining

Brucella anthracis

100

Streptococcus fecalis

1

Streptococcus hemolyticus

0.01

Staphylococcus aureus

0.0001

Streptococcus viridans

Staphylococcus albus

Diplococcus pneumoniae

—— Streptomycin —— Neomycin —— Penicillin

Figure 2.19 Mark Nicolich, Lambertville, NJ.

treatment of a malady caused by Gram-negative bacteria, Neomycin dominates. Even when it is not absolutely the best, it is so close to it that we can certainly live by the rule "Gram negative use Neomycin." When the bacteria are Gram positive the story is not quite so clear, but almost. Penicillin dominates except for two Staph and one Strep infection. Thus a treatment rule for Gram positive might be to use Penicillin and Neomycin in combination.

2.10 Conclusion

I have presented a lightning fast summary of data graphics using a single data source and showing a small sample of alternative methods for displaying them. This approach parallels, on a much smaller scale, Jacques Bertin's famous "100 bad examples" except that almost all of the alternatives included were pretty good. Many were marvelous. A more detailed story can be found in the standard works (listed in the references).

My focus here has been on trying to find a general purpose display that does a good job at answering all of the principal questions. Remarkably, there were a number of formats that accomplished this reasonably well; several beautifully. We are not always this lucky. Sometimes we must be satisfied with a display that answers one question well and, hopefully, leaves the vast darkness of the other questions unobscured.

Returning to the core topic of this section, evidence-based medicine, it is worth remembering that the definition of evidence is *data related to the question at issue.* Displaying data without a question is not evidence. As an example consider the display shown as Figure 2.20. This was prepared by Christine Schmotzer, a pathologist, who explained that in 1951 there was an emergence of new antibiotics and the central question that physicians asked was "what is this drug good for?" Her design, shown as Figure 2.20, answers this question clearly.

But if we want to look at the obverse question ("What's the best drug to control this Strep infection?") we have to search, making this display less valuable than an alphabetical table. In fact, for very specific questions, a sentence may be the most efficient answer. Thus for narrow purposes a highly specific display may be of great evidentiary value. But there are often multiple goals, one of which is often to have the data guide us to more interesting questions. In situations like these a more general display that answers multiple questions, is more valuable. And for hypothesis generation a display that serves us best is one that *forces* us

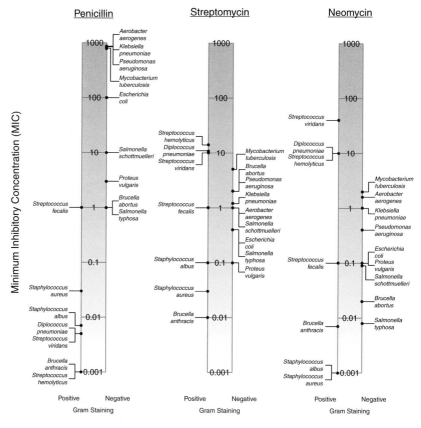

Figure 2.20 Christine Schmotzer, Pathology, Emory University.

to see what we were not expecting. Indeed, data graphs are the most powerful tools we have for doing this.

What have we learned from this exhibition of pictures?

1 There are many paths to salvation. For any data set there are many possible good displays, although the same rules for construction underlay them all.

2 Any display can be improved. Good writing means we rewrite our prose many times. Because images are more memorable than words, it is even more important to revise our displays than our words. In the past this was difficult and expensive. Now it isn't.

3 A display is never done—genius is the infinite capacity for taking pains.

4 Accurate interpretation of results often needs more information. For example, how does our interpretation of these results change when we learn that kidney damage sometimes accompanies the overuse of Neomycin? And, as we shall

learn in Chapter 3, we pay a large price if we do not try to understand the substantive material that the data represent. We need to be able to read the names of the bacteria and think about what their depiction in the plot might imply.

This brief introduction indicates some of the difficulties in the effective display of information as well as the enormous value of doing it well. To embrace evidence-based medicine we must also embrace looking at evidence effectively.[5] This exhibition of pictures provides a graphic case study of the many paths available as well as the rewards associated with doing it well.

It isn't hard to look at each of the displays presented here and think of small changes that might yield proportional improvements, but these are nits. The best of the displays here present a coherent, memorable picture of the data, and can scale upward to include more bacteria and more antibiotics. Will Burtin would be impressed.

CHAPTER 3

That's funny . . .

The most exciting phrase to hear in science. The one that heralds new discoveries, is not "Eureka" but "That's funny. . . . "

Isaac Asimov *(1920–1992)*

The Princeton polymath, John Tukey (1915–2000) observed "the greatest value of a graph is when it *forces* us to see what we never expected." Of course to allow the graph to develop its most forceful personality we must plot the data in an appropriate way. I will illustrate this with a powerful example of how valuable such a graphic design can prove to be when it is done well, and viewed through an appropriately quizzical lens[1].

Once again let us use the data that Will Burtin summarized in the 1951 display discussed in Chapter 2, showing the efficacy of three antibiotics on 16 different kinds of bacteria.

To ease comparisons I repeat the graphic that Burtin designed to depict these data in Figure 3.1 (previously Figure 2.3).

The display is divided into two sections depending on whether the bacteria in question were affected by a Gram stain or not. Burtin's display focuses on the efficacy of the antibiotics and, as we saw in Chapter 2, careful study of it reveals that if a bacteria is Gram positive it can be efficaciously treated with a combination of Penicillin and/or Neomycin; if it is Gram negative Neomycin is the treatment of choice. But Burtin's display does not allow us to compare bacteria easily. This is a fundamental problem in graphic display.

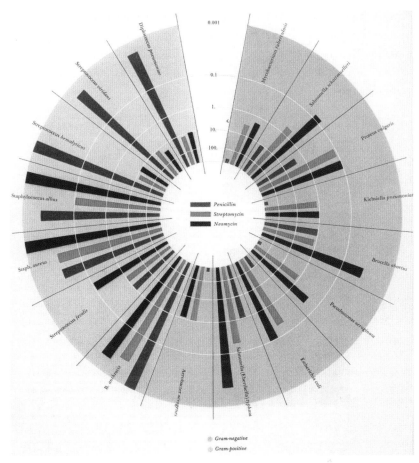

Burtin's diagram compares impacts of Penicillin, Streptomycin and Neomycin on a range of bacteria (*Scope*, Fall 1951). Copyright © Pfizer Inc. Reproduced with Permission.

Figure 3.1 Will Burtin's graphic depiction of the data from Table 2.1.
Antibacterial ranges of Neomycin, Penicillin and Streptomycin: The chart compares the in vitro sensitivities to Neomycin of some of the common pathogens (Gram-positive in red and Gram-negative in blue) with their sensitivities to Penicillin and Streptomycin. The effectiveness of the antibiotics is expressed as the highest dilution in μg/ml, which inhibits the test organism. High concentrations are inward from the periphery; consequently the length of the colored bar is proportional to the effectiveness.

We can think of the component data as a table made up of 16 bacteria and three antibiotics. The two kinds of questions that naturally arise are:

(i) How do the drugs compare with respect to their differential efficacy?

(ii) How do the bacteria group together with respect to how they react to the various antibiotics?

Burtin's display aims at the former much more than the latter. It is easy to see why each of these two questions requires a different construction (although sometimes a very clever display can provide ingress to both). Jacques Bertin's (1918–2010) example (shown in Figure 3.2) has become a canonical illustration of this dilemma.

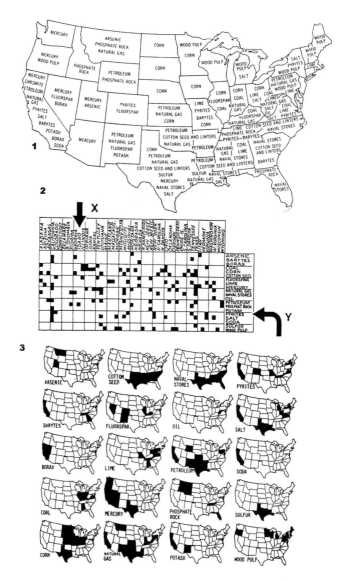

Figure 3.2 The canonical example of the two principal constructions from a typical data matrix from Jacques Bertin's *Graphics and the Graphical Treatment of Information* (1977).

The map at the top of the display (Panel 1) provides an answer to such questions as "What is produced in Nebraska?" A glance tells us corn. But if instead we were to ask the obverse question, "Where is corn produced?" this construction is of little use. To answer it we would need to look at every state and remember which ones produced corn. For questions of this latter type we would vastly prefer the compound construction at the bottom (panel 3), in which there is a separately shaded map for each product.

This emphasizes the importance of deciding what questions a display is to be answering, in advance of designing it. Obviously Burtin's choice was to compare drugs. As I show next, this has at least one unfortunate consequence.

If we were to focus on the task of comparing bacteria a different display might be more helpful. Let us reconsider the design previously shown as Figure 2.17, now, redrafted somewhat as Figure 3.3, in which each bacterium is given its own icon with little bars indicating how much of it was needed. The horizontal line depicts what might be considered the maximum plausible dosage, and so bars going down from that line depict clinically efficacious drugs.

Looking at this display, specifically at the row of bacteria resistant to Streptomycin and Neomycin, we see something funny. The pattern of response to the antibiotics of all three bacteria is essentially identical—two of these bacteria are Streptococcus and one is not. That seems odd. What is *Diplococcus pneumoniae* doing there? And, why does the third Strep bacteria, *Streptococcus faecalis* (in the next row up) appear to be so different? One would think that the genus of a bacterium would reflect similarities in what kills species that are members of that genus.

Because these oddities were not easily visible in Burtin's display, neither his, nor apparently anyone else's, curiosity was piqued. Had this odd structure been seen perhaps it would not have taken until 1974 for *Diplococcus pneumoniae* to be recognized as a Streptococcus and to be renamed *Streptococcus pneumoniae* (Howard & Gooder, 1974).

And why is *Streptococcus faecalis* so different? It would seem that its credentials as a member of the Strep family are impeccable; as Sherman, Mauer & Stark (1937, p. 275) described it:

In some respects Streptococcus faecalis (Andrewes & Horder, 1906) might be considered one of the better established species of the streptococci, and certainly some of the rather unique characteristics of this organism, or the general group to which it belongs, are commonly known by bacteriologists.

Yet, in 1984, its genus was changed and its name became *Enterococcus faecalis* (Schleifer & Kilpper-Balz, 1984). Perhaps had these data been plotted in a way that allowed us to compare the profile of responses of these various bacteria with

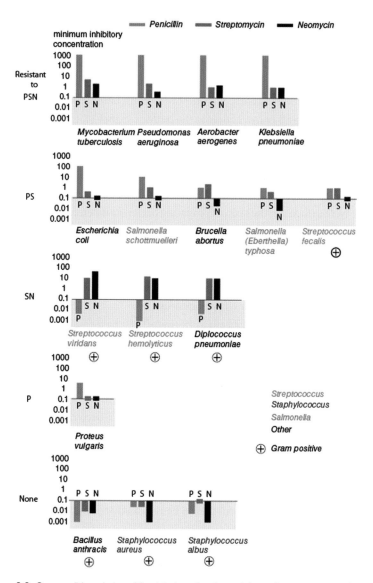

Figure 3.3 One possible redesign of Burtin's data, showing each bacterium as a separate icon with bars representing the log(MIC) for each antibiotic. It was originally designed by Brian Schmotzer of Emory University.

these antibiotics the classification of *Streptococcus faecalis* would have come under scrutiny sooner.

Remarkably, now that we know what to look for, it is easy to construct displays that show it. For example, a scatter plot of the performance of Penicillin vs. Neomycin (Figure 3.4) makes the clustering of *Diplococcus pneumoniae* with

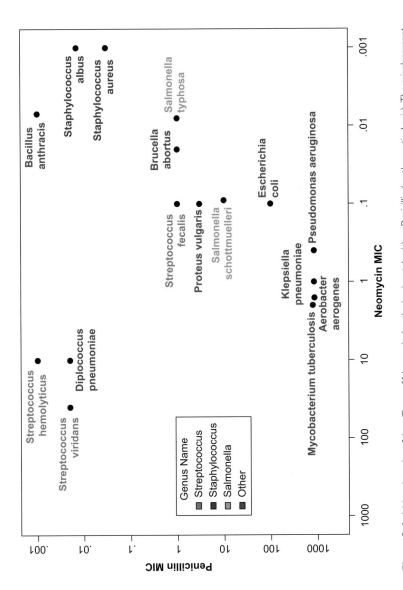

Figure 3.4 A bi-variate plot of the efficacy of Neomycin (on the horizontal axis) vs. Penicillin (on the vertical axis). The misplacement of two bacteria is obvious. Prepared by Shaun Lysen of the University of Pennsylvania.

the other two strep bacteria obvious, as is the distance between them and the incorrectly classified *Streptococcus faecalis*.

This investigation is meant only as one example of what could have been found if we had but taken the trouble to look. The early days of bacterial taxonomy had bacteria being classified using whatever tools were available: how they looked under the microscope, how they reacted to stains, etc. In 1951, when these data were published, antibiotics were relatively new and so using a bacterium's profile of reaction to them, while an obvious entry into their deep structure, was not yet a common tool. This demonstration shows what could have been found had the data been displayed properly. The classification using antibiotic reaction is now anachronistic for bacterial taxonomy; modern classification defines the relationships within genera by a unique RNA sequence (16S RNA) that is part of the bacterial ribosome. This sequence is like a finger-print for bacterial genera and species. But it is nice when some sort of phenotypic response confirms the tale told by the 16S RNA.

As we have discussed before, "Evidence-based science" is an ironic term; it does not mean that previous science was solely faith-based, although faith and the power of authority were certainly important prior to the modern desire to base decisions principally on empirical evidence. And having the epistemology of empiricism wasn't enough either. For if it was, the scientific method promulgated by Francis Bacon in the 16th century would not have taken 500 years to become dominant. Simply because a new idea is better is usually not enough, by itself, to allow it to supplant its predecessor. Samuel Johnson's quip on remarriage ("The triumph of hope over experience") generalizes beyond its original bounds. Too often we cling to outmoded theories despite accumulated evidence to the contrary (remember Galen's beautiful, but flawed, theory of the two-horned human uterus). I conclude this book (in Chapters 12 and 13) with five especially compelling additional examples of the difficulties faced in trying to overturn a mediocre convention even with a dramatically improved replacement.

But having a formal epistemological basis for evidence-based science was not enough; looking at evidence required effective methods for doing so. Language, developed long before science, was not an ideal match. Mathematics became the language of science but it too was ill-suited for looking at evidence. In the 17th century large tables of data were compiled, but this was not an answer; indeed two 19th century American economists emphasized the inadequacies of tabular presentation in their oft quoted quip,

Farquhar & Farquhar (*1891*)

And yet despite the warning of the brothers Farquahr, and the evidence of more than a century of scientific investigation, the table remains (by far) the principal means of communicating scientific evidence. In Figure 3.5 is a summary of the kinds of graphic forms used in a recent volume of the *Journal of the American Medical Association* (a similar picture would describe all of the other journals I have looked at). It is my view that this tabular approach is a mistake, for there is likely much that is being missed that might otherwise have been found.

Ironically, and in sharp contrast with our expectations based on the Farquahr's disdain for all that is tabular, a well-designed tabular display of Burtin's data tells us the same story, now that we know to look for it.

What lessons can we draw from this remarkable tale of discovery? It is evident that when data are displayed appropriately discoveries can be made that might have been missed. But there is more. The graph maker must have an appropriately prepared mind. Had we not cared about which data point represented which bacterium we would have missed everything. And this knowledge cannot

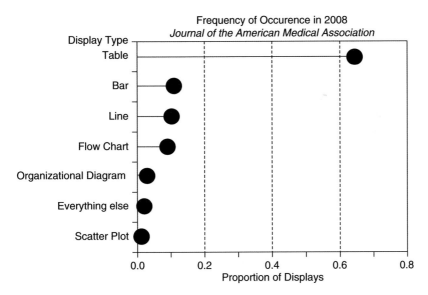

Figure 3.5 A dot plot showing the dominance of the Table in terms of its frequency of use vs. various other graphical forms in the 2008 volume of the *Journal of the American Medical Association*.

TABLE 3.1 A redesigned table of the Burtin data of the minimal inhibitory concentration (MIC) needed for three antibiotics on 16 bacteria ordered and spaced by the median MIC

Bacteria	Antibiotic			Gram staining	Row median
	Penicillin	Streptomycin	Neomycin		
Bacillis anthracis	−3.00	−2.00	−2.15	positive	−2.15
Staphylococcus albus	−2.15	−1.00	−3.00	positive	−2.15
Staphylococcus aureus	−1.52	−1.52	−3.00	positive	−1.52
Proteus *vulgaris*	0.48	−1.00	−1.00	negative	−1.00
Escherichia *coli*	2.00	−0.40	−1.00	negative	−0.40
Salmonella (Eberthella) *typhosa*	0.00	−0.40	−2.10	negative	−0.40
Salmonella *schottmuelleri*	1.00	−0.10	−1.05	negative	−0.10
Brucella *abortus*	0.00	0.30	−1.70	negative	0.00
Streptococcus *faecalis*	0.00	0.00	−1.00	positive	0.00
Klebsiella *pneumoniae*	2.93	0.08	0.00	negative	0.08
Aerobacter *aerogenes*	2.94	0.00	0.20	negative	0.20
Pseudomonas *aeruginosa*	2.93	0.30	−0.40	negative	0.30
Mycobacterium *tuberculosis*	2.90	0.70	0.30	negative	0.70
Diplococcus *pneumoniae*	−2.30	1.04	1.00	positive	1.00
Streptococcus *hemolyticus*	−3.00	1.15	1.00	positive	1.00
Streptococcus *viridans*	−2.30	1.00	1.60	positive	1.00

reside solely in the mind of the viewer of the graph, for without it the maker of the graph (if it is a different person) would have no guidance as to what it was that looked funny and thus might choose to present a final display that seemed pleasing on some other criteria. Being in a state of ignorance is rarely an advantage.

CHAPTER 4

Commentary on some graphs in the *2008 National Healthcare Quality Report*

4.1 Introduction

The healthcare of a nation's population is one of the most pressing issues for all governments. To do this efficiently and effectively requires keeping careful track of the outcomes of various alternative policies and practices. These issues were brought to the forefront of concern in the United States with the 2010 passage of the health care reform bill, for it is only in this way that we can assess the value of the legislation. It will also help to shape policy amendments in the future. Annually, there are many reports on various aspects of healthcare. The *2008 National Healthcare Quality Report*[1] represents the seventh annual version of what is a substantial effort to characterize some of the major questions about contemporary healthcare in the United States, to gather data that shed light on those questions, and to organize those data in a coherent and understandable form. This work was accomplished with considerable wisdom and many important decisions about inclusion, organization, and representation were made carefully and well. However, in any task as complex as this, improvements are always possible.

A fundamental tenet of quality control is that the improvement of any complex process is often best accomplished through the institution of an ongoing process of improvements. I strongly suspect that the seventh version of this report will not be the last, and so it seems worthwhile to take some time to suggest some improvements for future editions. These suggestions may have more general value, which has led me to offer these examples to a wider audience.

These suggestions are, to some extent, repetitious, for the same issues and hence solutions arose in Chapter 2. These duplications should be thought of as replication/validation, which is the sine qua non of science. It would be confusing indeed if the same problems that arose two chapters ago were dealt with differently now.

4.2 General display characteristics

The preparation of a chart book requires compromises. It is almost always better to choose a small number of conventional graphic formats and reuse them throughout than to invent unique display formats as the character of the data changes. Even though the latter approach may, in some sense, convey the special character of a particular data set, the cost to the reader of becoming familiar with a new format often outweighs any potential benefit. The *2008 National Healthcare Quality Report* (*2008 NHQR*) uses just three graphic formats—the line chart, the bar chart and the choropleth map—in combination with various kinds of tables, to convey their component data graphically. The decision to settle on but three formats seems wise to me, although the precise character of these representations can be improved.

Some principles upon which to improve graphic displays:

> I Goals must be clear and prioritized. To the four purposes I mentioned previously, exploration, communication, calculation and decoration, I would like to add a fifth: archiving—storing data for retrieval by others.

This purpose, although still considered, is now out of date, for there are far more convenient (typically electronic) modes of storing data that make retrieval and reorganization far easier.

Trying to accomplish too much usually impedes the efficacy of a display's primary purpose. For example, in this report the primary purpose is almost surely communication, but this is reduced when too many numbers are over-written on the graph in an effort to archive the data at the same time.

2 Scales should be chosen to match the purpose. The scales should be chosen to provide maximum acuity. In this way the viewer can often obtain quite an accurate sense of the component data without having to append the visual noise of numerical values. Too large a scale can hide real variations that then go unseen. Of course too small a scale can make random fluctuations seem real, but the viewer can always replot on the larger scale, an option that does not exist if the scale is too large. I view the "too small scale" as a venial sin, whereas the too large can be mortal.

3 Captions should be informative—there are two kinds of good graphs:

(i) strongly good graphs that tell you all you want to know just by looking at them; and

(ii) weakly good graphs that tell you all you want to know just by looking at them, once you know what to look for.

We can transform a weakly good graph into a strongly good one by having an informative/interpretive caption. Thus instead of a caption like "The rates of completion of tuberculosis treatment for different age groups" we might have "Although rates of completion of tuberculosis treatment have been increasing overall, children still have a 10% greater likelihood of completion than adults." By forcing the graph maker to include a caption on a display that explicitly tells the principal point of the display we gain two benefits; we can discover the point of the display more easily, and we lower the likelihood of pointless displays.

4 ALL is special and should be represented as such. Within any display it is often useful to represent some sort of summary measure—a mean, median, total—such a measure is different in kind from the various pieces that compose it. It is also more stable statistically by virtue of it being a composite measure. Thus its representation should be larger, darker and visually separate from the components.

5 Avoid legends whenever possible—a legend requires the viewer to first learn the legend and then apply it to the display; in Bertin's words, it requires two moments of perception and makes the viewer read the display rather than see it. A far better approach is to label the graphic elements directly.

6 We're almost never interested in "Alabama First"—the data elements should be ordered in a way that makes sense. Often ordering by size makes a coherent visual impact as well as suggesting an implicit underlying structure.

4.3 Examples from the *2008 NHQR*

Example 1. A bar chart

The first graph that we encounter in the summary section of the *NHQR* is a simple bar chart (Figure 4.1a), which was Figure H.1 in *NHQR*.

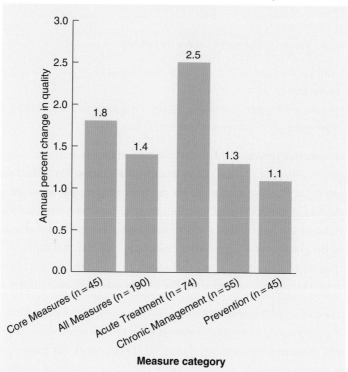

Figure H.1. Median annual rate of change overall and by measure category from baseline to most recent data year

Note: See Chapter 1, Introduction and Methods, for discussion of year intervals used for analysis. Ns indicate number of measures included in each group.

Figure 4.1a

Bar charts have a long history, but perceptual experiments have provided evidence that they can be improved. This one has a too-general label on the vertical axis. These data do not simply represent change; they represent improvement, for when the change is in the other direction the bar is directed downward. Thus the label ought to reflect this—*Annual percent improvement*.

Second, each bar has a long label, which is more easily read if it is written horizontally. This is best accomplished by turning the plot on its side.

Third, ALL needs to be visually emphasized and segregated.

Fourth, the inclusion of the actual percentages is redundant and adds more clutter than precision.

Fifth, ordering the categories by the extent of their improvement immediately aids our understanding of the relative rates of improvement, which seems to follow the path of triage—the most critical is improving the fastest.

And finally, the bar itself serves no purpose but to hold up the top line, which is the graphic element that conveys all of the information. By replacing the bar with a large dot at its top-most point we carry all the information but leave more room on the chart for additional material. To ease interpretation one can connect the dot to its identifying label with a thin line. An alternative version that makes these changes is shown in Figure 4.1b.

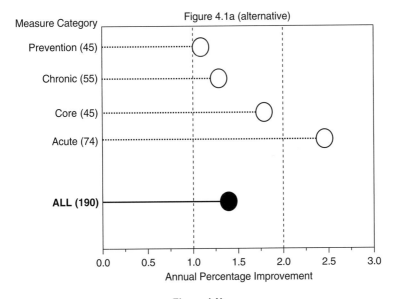

Figure 4.1b

The connecting line can be partially replaced by letting the label serve double duty and thus provide still more space as shown in the slightly modified version in Figure 4.1c.

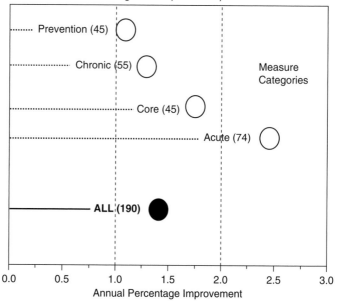

Figure 4.1a (alternative)

Figure 4.1c

Note that in both redesigns ALL is recognized as different and is so displayed. It is more vivid and spaced apart to perceptually accentuate its differentness.

The data are ordered rationally (almost surely not alphabetically). In this, as in most other situations ordering by size is effective.

As predicted, orienting the display horizontally rather than vertically has allowed the labels on each data point to be horizontal and hence read more easily.

The label on the x-axis is the more informative one. Accuracy in both words and numbers is important.

Last, removing the numerical values from the plot removes their visual clutter without subtracting useful information. If the plot is scaled properly the viewer can estimate the data value accurately enough. The report did not include the standard errors of the percentages, and so it was not obvious that the data were accurate to the nearest tenth of a percent. It is always wise not to portray data to any more precision than they are worth.

I believe that future designs should consider substituting the dot plot for the bar chart, when suitable. In the next example a different alternative is recommended for some bar charts.

Example 2. Another bar chart

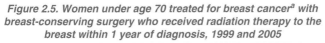

Figure 2.5. Women under age 70 treated for breast cancer[a] with breast-conserving surgery who received radiation therapy to the breast within 1 year of diagnosis, 1999 and 2005

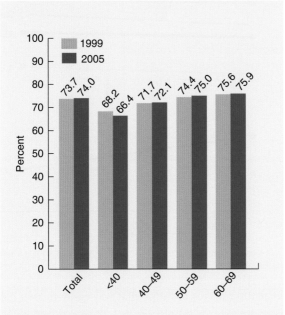

[a]American Joint Committee on Cancer Stage I, II, or III, primary invasive epithelial breast cancer.
Source: Commission on Cancer, American College of Surgeons and American Cancer Society, National Cancer Data Base, 1999 and 2005.
Reference population: U.S. population, women.

Figure 4.2a

This display (Figure 4.2a, which was Figure 2.5 in *NHQR*) shares some of the flaws of the previous one, and adds a new one; it represents a continuous variable, time, as different colored bars. Convention and good sense would suggest representing time on the x-axis with each of the age groups as separate graphical elements. This has the added advantage of scalability, so that when new time periods are available the plot can accommodate them effortlessly.

In the alternative below the format is changed to a line chart, with time on the x-axis. The vertical scale is expanded so that we can read off the specific values with enough accuracy to allow us to elide the distracting numerical barnacles. ALL is represented in a more dominant form, and the graphic elements that represent the various age groups are labeled directly.

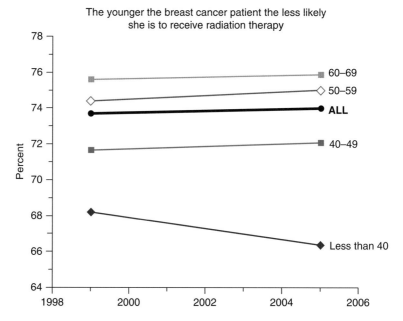

Figure 4.2b Data are the percentage of women, under the age of 70, treated for breast cancer with breast-conserving surgery who received radiation therapy to the breast within one year of diagnosis.

This representation makes obvious what was easily missed before—young women are very different. To emphasize this, the figure caption is modified to inform the viewer of the principal inferences that we are led to by these data.

Last, we note that there is a decline in the use of radiation between 1999 and 2005 for women under 40, yet all other groups increase, albeit slightly.

It might be useful, if we wish to make inferences about the changes in the use of radiation among breast cancer patients over time, to compute a value for ALL ages that is standardized to a fixed age population[2].

Example 3. Bars for time, again

I want to emphasize the point that bars on a time chart do not usually work as well as other formats (Figure 4.3a, which was Figure 2.1 in *NHQR*). A line chart uses less graphical space than a bar and provides a more evocative metaphor. Again, by avoiding legends as much as possible we can see the display rather than having to read it. It is always preferred, if possible, to label the data representation directly rather than through a legend. This is not always possible, but when it is, it should be done this way. The vertical axis is labeled a bit more fully than just the almost worthless "percent." And last, ALL is treated differently, as befitting its special character (Figure 4.3b).

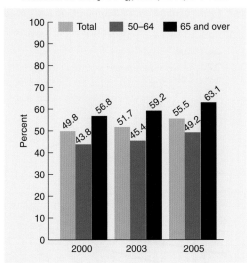

Figure 2.1. Adults age 50 and over who ever received colorectal cancer screening (colonoscopy, sigmoidoscopy, proctoscopy, or fecal occult blood test [FOBT]), 2000, 2003, and 2005

Source: Centers for Disease Control and Prevention, National Center for Health Statistics, National Health Interview Survey, 2000, 2003, and 2005.
Reference population: Civilian noninstitutionalized population age 50 and over.
Note: Total rate is adjusted to the 2000 U.S. standard population.

Figure 4.3a

Note that this format will scale easily to include many more years, as well as additional age groups, whereas the bar chart format quickly becomes hopelessly jumbled.

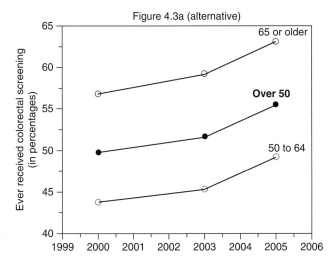

Figure 4.3b

Example 4. A line chart that not even a mother could love

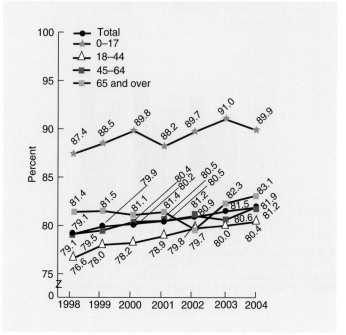

Figure 2.39. Patients with tuberculosis who completed acurative course of treatment within 1 year of initiation of treatment, by age group, 1998–2004

Source: Centers for Disease Control and Prevention, National Tuberculosis Surveillance System, 1998–2004.
Reference population: U.S. civilian noninstitutionalized population.

Figure 4.4a

Not all lines charts representing time are winners. Figure 4.4a (which was Figure 2.39 in *NHQR*) is a complex mess made so through the mistaken insistence that all data values be included and the various graphical elements be identified through a legend. A naïve viewing of this plot might suggest that the complexity of the visual experience is inescapably part of the complexity of the underlying phenomenon. But is this true?

In the alternative sketched in Figure 4.4b I have expanded the scale on the vertical axis so we can estimate the individual data values with enough accuracy for most purposes and expanded the axis label to be more fully descriptive. I replaced the legend and labeled each line directly, and last, made the figure caption more descriptive, to inform the viewer of the key aspects of the data. Obviously, the details of the groups being plotted must still be included, but they can occupy a less dominant position on the chart, akin to a footnote.

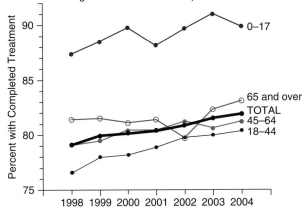

Figure 4.4a (alternative). Although rates of completion of tuberculosis treatment have been increasing overall, children still have a 10% greater likelihood of completion than adults.

Figure 4.4b

This chart is for patients with tuberculosis who completed a curative course of treatment within one year of initiation of treatment, by age group, 1998–2004.

Example 5. A line chart with a linear extrapolation

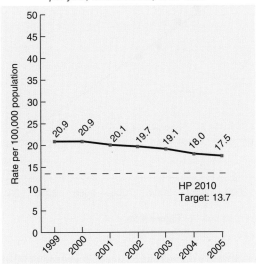

Figure 2.4. Colorectal cancer deaths per 100,000 population per year, United States, 1999–2005

Source: Centers for Disease Control and Prevention, National Center for Health Statistics, National Vital Statistics System-Mortality, 1999–2005.
Reference population: U.S. population.
Note: Age adjusted to the 2000 U.S. standard population. Healthy People 2010 target is revised. Please see Chapter 1, Introduction and Methods, for details.

Figure 4.5a

Figure 4.5a (which was Figure 2.4 in *NHQR*) is a simple, straightforward plot. There are only seven data points and so it would take heroic efforts to make them incomprehensible. The data are so simple that a line chart of them can absorb some of the flaws of the other line charts (e.g. a too large scale, inclusion of data values) without serious ill effects. But the *NHQR* uses the data from this display to make a prediction. It concludes, "At the present rate of change from 1999 to 2005, this target (a colorectal cancer death rate of 13.7 per 100,000) will not be met by 2010."

Figure 4.5a can be improved in a number of small ways that were illustrated in the previous examples. If the y-axis scale is expanded to cover only 12–22% we can read off the data entries without having to write them in. We can expand the time axis to 2012 to show how the linear extrapolation will intersect the goal for 2010 about a year late. We also can insert the fitted equation to emphasize that the rate of colorectal cancer mortality is shrinking by about 0.6% per year (obtained from the slope of the fitted line) (Figure 4.5b).

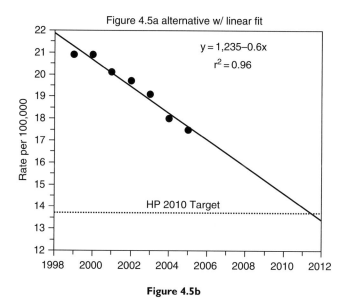

Figure 4.5b

But extrapolation is always a dangerous business. If instead of fitting the data with a linear function suppose we fit a quadratic function (which fits even better) we would find that we make the target date with room to spare (Figure 4.5c). It is probably wise to explicitly state what the extrapolating assumptions are before announcing a prediction. Also just saying that the target will not be met is less helpful than pointing out exactly when our extrapolation predicts that it would be reached.

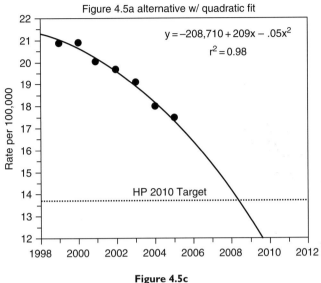

Figure 4.5a alternative w/ quadratic fit

$$y = -208,710 + 209x - .05x^2$$
$$r^2 = 0.98$$

HP 2010 Target

Figure 4.5c

Example 6. A choropleth map

When data are gathered from various geographic areas a common method for displaying them is the choropleth map, in which the geographic entities are shaded in a way that represents the data values that were generated by that region. Figure 4.6 (which was Figure 2.2 in *NHQR*) is a typical choropleth map that has the virtues and flaws of all such displays. It provides a bit of visual distortion since the size of the state, and hence its visual impact, often has little relationship to the underlying variable of interest (e.g. population size). This flaw is dramatically displayed on election nights when big sparsely populated states are all red and small, densely populated ones are blue. A naïve look would strongly suggest a red victory, even when it was a blue landslide. But this is the price we must pay for the benefits of such a display (showing the location of the phenomenon being plotted).

This plot, and others like it, could be improved by using a shading metaphor that is ordered. The current scheme is not helpful. There is no way to know (without the legend) that black is high and blue is low and green is average. Instead, if we used a naturally ordered metaphor, the result would be easier to

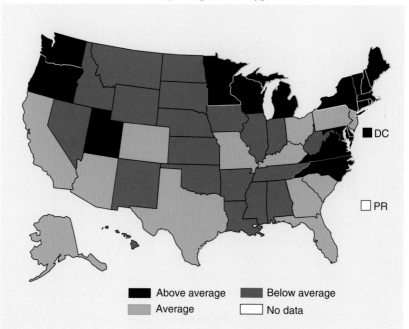

Figure 2.2. State variation: Adults age 50 and over who ever received a colonoscopy or sigmoidoscopy, 2006

Legend:
- Above average
- Below average
- Average
- No data

Key: Above average = rate in significantly above the reporting States average in 2006. Below average = rate is significantly below the reporting States average in 2006.
Source: Centers for Disease Control and Prevention, Behavioral Risk Factor Surveillance System, 2006.
Note: Age adjusted to the 2000 U.S. standard population. The "reporting States average" is the average of all reporting States (51 in this case, including the District of Columbia), which is a separate figure form the national average. Data source differs form national estimates in Figure 2.1. Figure does not include proctoscopy or fecal occult blood test.

Figure 4.6

see. One way, in a monochrome display, is to use "darker = more." If you wanted to use color it would be with increasing saturations. Note that this method easily scales to more than three categories; indeed we could use continuous shading and not need to use such a coarse categorization as "below average," "above average" and "average." We could actually shade according to the amount and then provide a legend that pairs a scale (say 40 to 75) with the associated shading. We could even use such a method on much smaller geographic entities (e.g. counties or census tracts) and, with suitable smoothing, be able to spot phenomena that are related to, say, urban vs. rural, rather than state by state.[3]

Also it is wasteful to use a single category for only one territory. A line of prose works far better. One alternative could be:

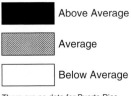

There are no data for Puerto Rico

4.4 Discussion and conclusions

This is an especially important time to work hard on accurately measuring the efficacy of healthcare in the United States, for we are on the brink of a major change in the way healthcare is delivered and paid for. It is crucial to know the extent to which these changes have accomplished their goal of increasing access to medical care and thence improving the length and quality of Americans' lives.

The existing reports have done much of the hard work of deciding what topics would be included, collecting the data that illuminate those topics, and deciding how they would be organized. In this chapter I have tried to provide some suggestions as to how the reporting might be improved.

We have seen how the same few principles that generated clear avenues for improvement in the plots of the antibiotic data in Chapters 2 and 3 applied in these charts as well. These are general rules that ought to be applied widely. In addition, I would like to emphasize the value of replacing the bar chart format with dot charts. Aside from their cleaner look, there is substantial experimental evidence[4] that they perform better. I also believe that it would be wise to abandon the practice of redundantly including the value of all data points on each graph. If such information is deemed to be important to convey to the reader, place them in associated tables in an appendix, or better, as EXCEL files on a web-site.

CHAPTER 5

Improving graphic displays by controlling creativity

Those who cannot remember the past are condemned to repeat it.

George Santayana *(1863–1952)*

5.1 Introduction

I could not help but think of George Santayana's observation on the importance of knowing the past while I was studying the New York State cancer maps discussed in Chapter 1. Or, more specifically, the legislation's insistence on the presentation of the raw/unadjusted cancer data. As I illustrated in that earlier discussion, the depiction of such data is a misinterpretation waiting to happen. What is sad is that we know better, and, we have known better for a long time.

In May of 1998, the revered polymath John Tukey wrote a 12-page letter to Linda Pickle. The letter was his response to *The Atlas of United States Mortality* (1996) that Dr. Pickle and her colleagues at the National Center for Health Statistics had published. He said "It is by far the best job of this sort that I have seen. It probably deserves a grade of between 94 and 98 out of 100." He then spent the rest of his note with suggestions for improvement. But before he turned to those suggestions he added,

Things like "*The Atlas*" evolve over a substantial period of time and I have no reason to believe that a document responsive to the emendations that follow (be they good or bad) would represent the end of the evolutionary process. Whatever the next step of advance may be, once taken, will, I trust with near certainty, open up our thinking to new possibilities beyond those we have so far imagined.

These are wise words indeed and suggest a pathway of evolution for statistical reports in which the direction of improvement is likely to be monotonic, with only small local variants.

I will not attempt to describe all of the design decisions that went into *The Atlas* that Tukey gave such high grades, but instead recommend to all who have not yet had the pleasure, to immediately run out and get a copy of their own. I will, however, focus on one characteristic of that fine report, germane to my topic. Specifically, improving the quality of a report through the tight control of creativity.

Example 1. *The Atlas of Mortality*

The *Atlas* has a very regular structure. Its body is made up of 18 sections, each concerned with mortality from a specific cause (e.g. cancer, stroke, motor vehicle injuries, diabetes, firearms, etc.). Then each section, in its turn, is sub-divided into four sections corresponding to white females, black females, white males, and black males. Each of those is composed of a large colored map whose HSAs (Health Service Areas) are shaded and colored to represent the age-adjusted death rates for that cause and that demographic group. On the facing page are three smaller maps showing the variations for age 40 and another for age 70 and the third showing a comparison of the death rates compared with the overall US rate. There is also a small plot showing regional variation. The first chapter of the *Atlas* goes over this format, carefully explaining as well the various statistical adjustments and smoothings that yielded the figures presented.

Obviously an enormous amount of attention went into the basic design and, I assume, what we see is the result of endless discussions and compromises. Once the design was set it was then repeated exactly from chapter to chapter. This makes it easier on the reader who has only to master the design once and can then read it through with no further education. *The Atlas* accomplishes this so gracefully that the reader can be blissfully unaware of how hard it must have been to control rampant creativity[1]. I am sure that someone must've argued desperately to use a histogram made up of miniature Colt 45s to indicate firearms

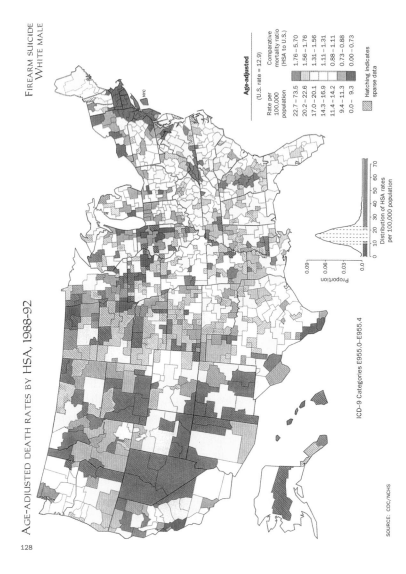

AGE-ADJUSTED DEATH RATES BY HSA, 1988-92

FIREARM SUICIDE
WHITE MALE

Age-adjusted

Rate per 100,000 population	Comparative mortality ratio (HSA to U.S.)
(U.S. rate = 12.9)	
22.7 – 73.5	1.76 – 5.70
20.2 – 22.6	1.56 – 1.76
17.0 – 20.1	1.31 – 1.56
14.3 – 16.9	1.11 – 1.31
11.4 – 14.2	0.88 – 1.11
9.4 – 11.3	0.73 – 0.88
0.0 – 9.3	0.00 – 0.73

Hatching indicates sparse data

Proportion

0.09
0.06
0.03
0.0

0 10 20 30 40 50 60 70
Distribution of HSA rates per 100,000 population

ICD–9 Categories E955.0–E955.4

SOURCE: CDC/NCHS

Figure 5.1 Age-adjusted death rates for Firearm suicides for white males, 1988–1992, from Pickle et al. (1996). These displays were on facing pages and constituted the standard format for the entire *Atlas*.

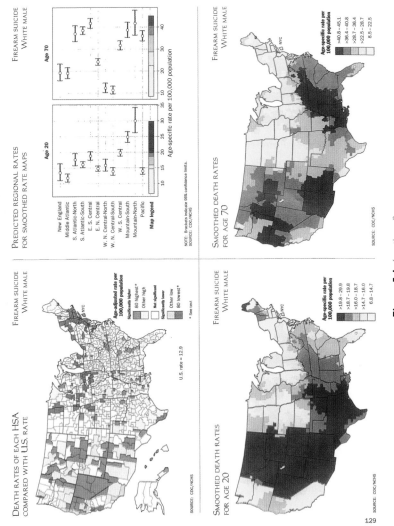

DEATH RATES OF EACH HSA
COMPARED WITH U.S. RATE

FIREARM SUICIDE
WHITE MALE

PREDICTED REGIONAL RATES
FOR SMOOTHED RATE MAPS

FIREARM SUICIDE
WHITE MALE

Age 20

Age 70

New England
Middle Atlantic
S. Atlantic-North
S. Atlantic-South
E. S. Central
E. N. Central
W. N. Central-North
W. N. Central-South
W. S. Central
Mountain-South
Mountain-North
Pacific

Map legend

Age-specific rate per 100,000 population

NOTE: Brackets indicate 95% confidence limits.
SOURCE: CDC/NCHS

Age-adjusted rate per
100,000 population

Significantly higher
80 highest*
Other high
Not significant
Significantly lower
Other low
80 lowest*

* See text

U.S. rate = 12.9

SOURCE: CDC/NCHS

SMOOTHED DEATH RATES
FOR AGE 20

FIREARM SUICIDE
WHITE MALE

SMOOTHED DEATH RATES
FOR AGE 70

FIREARM SUICIDE
WHITE MALE

Age-specific rate per
100,000 population

>19.8 – 29.9
>18.7 – 19.8
>16.0 – 18.7
>14.7 – 16.0
6.8 – 14.7

SOURCE: CDC/NCHS

Age-specific rate per
100,000 population

>40.8 – 45.1
>36.4 – 40.8
>28.7 – 36.4
>22.5 – 28.7
8.5 – 22.5

SOURCE: CDC/NCHS

Figure 5.1 (continued).

129

deaths. But happily editorial wisdom has shaded our eyes from such creative brilliance.

When we choose a display format there can be competing forces. On the one hand we may invent a specific format that conforms exactly to the data and to the demands associated with communicating the message contained within those data, yet such a format would be foreign to the audience. On the other hand there may be a standard format, familiar to the readers that does the job almost as well. Which do we choose? Convention is very powerful and unless the gains from defying convention are monstrous, it is usually a mistake to opt for the innovative. The odds change, however, if we are designing an extensive statistical report in which we have the opportunity to reuse the unconventional display often. In this situation it may be worth the reader's time to learn the new format. *The Atlas* uses a moderately unusual display format, but it is only new the first time.

The earliest example I know of how quickly people can learn is an early bar chart. Joseph Priestley's 1765 plot (see Figure 5.2) of the lives of famous men in history[2]. When it first appeared it was accompanied by several pages of textual description, ostensibly to help the reader who had surely never seen anything like it before. Yet in his 1769 elaboration Priestley included essentially no further explanation.

Example 2. *Understanding USA*

But stifling creative urges has obviously been too difficult, even at the cost of reducing the effectiveness of communication, for some authors. For example in *Understanding USA*, a chart book put out by the Markle Foundation, every page uses a different display format. The only thing they seem to have in common is that they are all mostly indecipherable. I believe that if they had followed the path provided by Linda Pickle and her colleagues in their *Atlas* and agreed to a common graphical format it would have solved two problems. Obviously the problem of deciphering a new format on each page would disappear, but also if each proponent of a particular format had to convince the other authors/designers of its efficacy the weaknesses of that format would be exposed and corrected. Moreover, by finding a general format, suitable for a broad range of data, simplicity would surely have trumped chartjunk. I include, as Figure 5.3, one example from a chapter by Hani Rashid and Lise Ann Couture. As hard as this may be to believe, this display is not notably worse than many of the others contained in this remarkable volume.

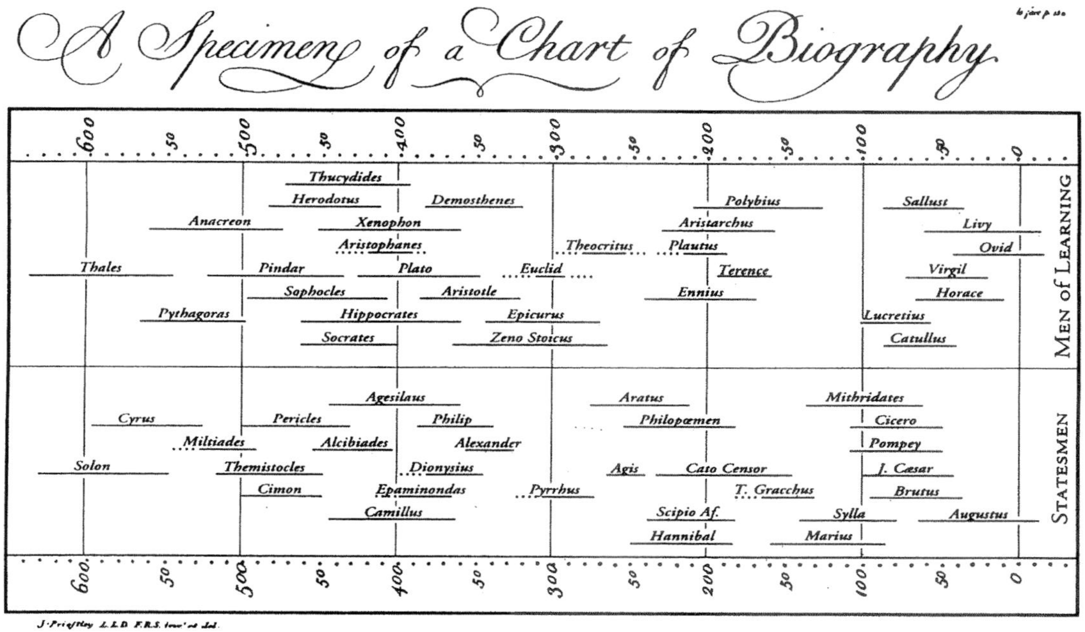

A Specimen of a Chart of Biography.

Men of Learning

Statesmen

Men of Learning: Sallust, Livy, Ovid, Virgil, Horace, Lucretius, Catullus, Polybius, Aristarchus, Plautus, Terence, Ennius, Theocritus, Euclid, Epicurus, Zeno Stoics, Demosthenes, Xenophon, Aristophanes, Plato, Aristotle, Thucydides, Herodotus, Hippocrates, Socrates, Pindar, Sophocles, Anacreon, Thales, Pythagoras

Statesmen: Mithridates, Cicero, Pompey, J. Cæsar, Brutus, Sylla, Marius, Augustus, Aratus, Philopœmen, Agis, Cato Censor, T. Gracchus, Scipio Af., Hannibal, Pyrrhus, Agesilaus, Philip, Alexander, Alcibiades, Dionysius, Epaminondas, Camillus, Pericles, Themistocles, Cimon, Miltiades, Cyrus, Solon

J. Priestley LL.D. F.R.S. inv. et del.

Figure 5.2 Joseph Priestley's chart of biography from his 1765 publication. See Wainer (2005) Chapter 5 for a fuller description of it.

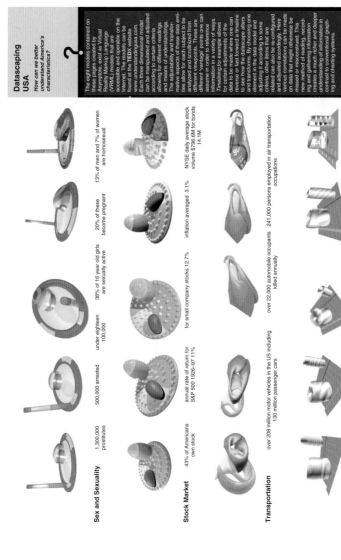

Figure 5.3 An incomprehensible plot of some unrelated things, from Wurman (2000).

Example 3. *Cancer Trends Report*

On December 12, 2007 the US National Cancer Institute provided their annual *Cancer Trends Progress Report*[3]. In it they followed the model provided by Linda Pickle and her colleagues a decade earlier. Each chapter frames some questions about cancer, its detection and its risk factors, and then caps the questions with various sound-bite-suitable responses. Each section then culminates with a graph. The graphical format is simple and clear and always the same (see Figure 5.4). The figures are apparently produced in some automatic way and so some unfortunate choices of color and label placement get made, perhaps by accident (or perhaps by an imperfect algorithm). However, even though the figure is reasonably clear there are still some improvements that can be made. And so in the spirit of Tukey's suggestions a decade ago let me offer ten suggestions (implemented in Figure 5.5), so that future versions of this report will be still

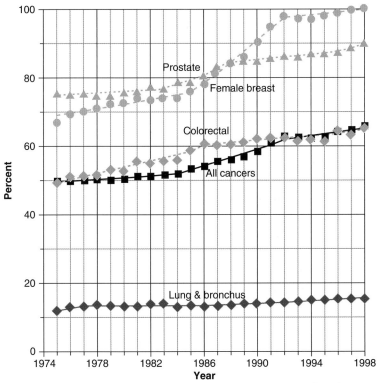

Source: SEER Program, National Cancer Institute. Rates are from the SEER 9 areas (http://seer.cancer.gov/registries/terms.html).\
Data are not age-adjusted.

Figure 5.4 Five-year survival rates from various kinds of cancer showing the improvements over the last two decades; from National Cancer Institute report.

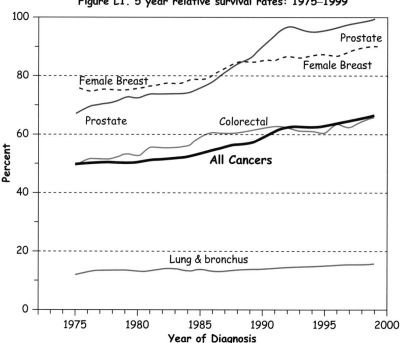

Figure L1. 5 year relative survival rates: 1975–1999

Percent

Year of Diagnosis

Figure 5.5 Figure 5.4 redrafted with ten changes.

better and, more generally, that the original paired with the revision can serve as an guide for all who construct displays. I don't labor under the misapprehension that the revisions I am proposing are the end of the line, but only that they correct some flaws and might suggest further avenues for progress.

1 Obviously, light colors (like yellow) should be avoided, as their visibility is easily compromised. Moreover, not all users of a report will have easy access to color printing, and so it is important, when possible, for all the colors used to be completely readable if the plot is to be reproduced in black and white.

2 When lines cross ambiguity is reduced if both ends are labeled.

3 Axes should be spaced logically. In this instance, why should the x-axis be spaced in 4-year intervals? Such a convention makes sense if the phenomenon being plotted happens at four-year intervals (e.g. US presidential elections). Otherwise it is sensible to stay with the convention of five or ten year intervals, which are derivative of our base-ten society. It is especially suitable for these data to emphasize the five-year survival criterion.

4 Labels must be large enough to be easily read and positioned so as not to have their referent be confused.

5 Once again, the category "ALL" is special—it should be made darker and bigger to differentiate it from its components.

6 The x-axis label should be made both complete and explicit—the partial label "year" is ambiguous. It could be the year of diagnosis (my guess) or the year that the survey noted the patient was still alive.

7 Too many extra grid lines add little but visual noise. They should be omitted if their loss yields no loss of information. I sketched in just four major horizontal lines to aid orientation (e.g. lung cancer five-year survival rates are less than 20%) and to add extra horizontal references that emphasize the gentle positive slopes for all the curves (even lung cancer) that constitute some of the good news contained in the report.

8 There should be some space between the axes and the first and last data points so that no points are obscured by sitting on an axis.

9 Plotting points can be deleted once they serve their purpose of showing where the connecting function needs to go. Leaving them in is like leaving up the scaffolding after a building is complete.

10 A friendlier font than Helvetica may be found less off-putting to readers. Helvetica is a clean, austere, serious-looking font; it is frequently a good choice. But a document focusing on cancer does not need anything extra to impress its seriousness on the reader. A little visual gentleness may serve us well.

5.2 Conclusions

The lessons to be learned from these three examples are simple:

(i) The path to improved display is endless, but mostly monotonic, if we learn from the past and continue to innovate, standing on the shoulders of our predecessors.

(ii) Innovation should be controlled; too much may increase the load on the viewers beyond their capacity. Also the graphical inventors of the past were not idiots, and the inventions that have survived time have done so because of their usefulness over a broad range of areas of application. It is possible that we can invent something entirely new and superior to all that has come before, but the odds are against it. Minard did, but such ideas don't come along all that often, which is why we still celebrate his flow maps more than a century later. Control hubris.

(iii) When trying to prepare a coherent report on a single, possibly broad, topic the displays should be coherent as well. Repeating the same format with different data eases the decoding task of the viewer. It is usually a mistake to think that such repetitiveness will bore the readers; quite the opposite. It will allow them to focus on the content of the displays and not their format. In the end they will be grateful.

(iv) A complex statistical report often has many authors, each preparing a separate section. If only a single presentation format is to be used throughout, there must be considerable cooperation among the authors and strong leadership from the editor. The multiple eyes and minds looking at each section that this approach requires is almost sure to lead to improved quality. It is an important benefit of cooperation[4].

Some Advances

It is easy to lie with statistics, but easier to lie without them.

Frederick Mosteller

Introduction

The study of the Science of Statistics has been replacing the study of calculus as universi-ties' principal required course in the mathematical sciences. This action has grown more popular as the realization has spread that it is more important for a literate citizen of the modern world to develop facility in statistical thinking than to understand the mathemat-ics of infinitesimals.

In Chapters 6 through 11 I illustrate how statistical thinking combined with graphical display allows us to make progress on some important issues.

Chapter 6 confronts the problem of living with a chronic disease, in this case diabetes. Diabetes must be dealt with 24 hours a day, every day, but typical diabetics see their physician for only a few hours every year. In this chapter I examine how we can use the data gathered by, and stored in, a diabetic's glucose meter to provide help in managing the disease.

Chapter 7 is about improving the diagnostic accuracy of X-rays of hip fractures. Not all orthopedic surgeons are equally aggressive in recommending major surgery to repair a hip fracture. In this chapter I show how adjusting for this differential aggressiveness improves the accuracy of diagnosis, and speculate on how this adjustment may affect patient decisions.

In Chapter 8 I tell an important and surprising story about probability. The principal area of discussion is on the divisive topic of the value of mammograms in improving women's lives. I take the opportunity to show the similarity between this topic and find-ing terrorists. In it, you will learn the apparently paradoxical fact that, although a mam-mogram will detect a tumor, if it is there, nine times out of ten, if it does say there is a tumor only one time in twenty will this be correct. Once we understand this we begin to understand why there are so many innocent people in prison.

Predicting the future from the past is a better option than predicting on the basis of no information at all, but it carries with it very real dangers. In *Life on the Mississippi*, Mark Twain noted how the Mississippi River, by cutting across meanders, has periodically shortened itself in the past. From this he deduced that it must've been more than a million miles long in the old Oolithic Silurian period "just a million years ago next November" when it must have "stuck out over the Gulf of Mexico like a fishing pole." Then looking forward he predicted that in the 21st century the Mississippi River would be just a mile and a quarter long and the streets of Cairo (Illinois) and New Orleans would be joined and the two cities would be stumbling along comfortably with a single mayor and board of aldermen. He concluded that this is what he loved about science, "with such a small investment of fact we can gather huge dividends of conjecture." Yet sometimes we must predict the future and all we have to go on is the past and present. In Chapter 9 we explore how one might predict the long-term effects of medical treatments when all we have to work with are short-term data.

Chapter 10 continues in our investigation of medical predictions. In this instance we look at predictions made by psychiatrists about the future behavior of criminals. We learn that both sides of an argument among psychiatrists about the probity of convicted felons were wrong and grew from a lack of understanding probability and loss functions. Samuel Johnson's horse provides us with a useful orienting attitude.

Chapter 11 concludes this section by trying to unravel the vexing mystery surrounding the shrinking efficacy of medical treatments as we study them more fully. But just as clarity starts to be manifest, we are confronted with conflicting results from Chinese medical researchers that fly in the face of all that we thought we knew. In the end we can only conclude that medical research should join with toys and drywall on the list of things we ought not to import from China.

Diabetes and the obesity epidemic: Taking a better look at blood sugar as a start

6.1 Introduction

It is estimated that there are 23.6 million children and adults in the United States, or almost 8% of the population, who have diabetes[1]. Of these 16.9 million have been diagnosed and 5.7 million people (or nearly one-third) are unaware that they have the disease[2]. The large proportion of undiagnosed diabetics adds some uncertainty to the estimates of the total number, but through the use of multiple sources and some statistical adjustment we can obtain a rough view (see Figure 6.1). Using adjusted estimates of the prevalence of this disorder we can see that over the past 70 years the growth of diabetes in the US has been exponential. There have been many causes proposed for this explosion including increasing obesity, decreasing physical activity, a shifting of diet toward more processed foods, and an aging population. There are many other risk factors, the exploration of which is not the principal purpose of this chapter. Instead I would like to focus on making the treatment of the disease more efficacious through improved communication of the consequences of treatment choices and behaviors.

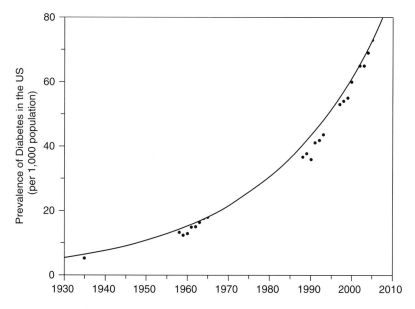

Figure 6.1 Estimates of the prevalence of diabetes in the US shown as the number per 1,000 in the population. The fitted curve is an exponential function.

Although dealing with diabetes more effectively is certainly an important enough topic to justify its own chapter, it seems worthwhile to be explicit about how improvements in communicating health status/blood sugar to diabetics can generalize to allied topics. Specifically, the growing obesity of the developed world's populace is both a contributing factor to the growth of diabetes and to many other health issues (e.g. heart disease, skeletal problems). I believe that the recommendations that emerge from this chapter can provide help to those who want to control their weight better.

Left untreated, diabetes has many serious consequences including, but not restricted to, liver and kidney damage, and circulatory problems leading to blindness, neuropathy, and loss of limbs. But effective treatment requires close cooperation between the physician and the patient. The physician can prescribe drugs and changes in diet and exercise regimes, but only the patient can implement those changes. Often the patient is given both general and specific guidelines, but the effects of following, or not following those guidelines can only be seen after implementation. The record of success cannot be described as an unqualified one. Indeed, as RAND scientist Jinan Saaddine explains, "Despite the many improvements, 2 in 5 people with diabetes still have poor cholesterol control, 1 in 3 have poor blood pressure control, 1 in 5 have poor glucose control." Why? Surely the consequences of not controlling cholesterol, glucose and blood pressure are both dire and clearly understood. Just as surely, the answer to the causal "why?' has many parts. We would like to consider just one of them here: the communication of current status to the patient is not as effective as it could be.

6.2 What is

Once a patient is diagnosed with diabetes a number of actions take place. Among them are extensive counseling about the importance of keeping blood sugar under tight control and the role that diet and exercise play in so doing. To aid the patient in controlling blood sugar she or he is given a small device that (i) reads a small blood sample and indicates its glucose content within seconds, (ii) records the reading along with the time and date it was taken, (iii) allows the inputting of various classifying characteristics (e.g. before a meal, after a meal, or none), (iv) calculates mean blood sugar levels for the last 7 days, 14 days and 30 days, and (v) shows these averages for each of the sub classifications indicated in (iii). All in all, this small instrument is a remarkable device.

As remarkable as this device is, with a few minor modifications it could be more useful still by (a) modifying how it summarizes the data, and (b) how it displays them. My suggestions on how to improve matters is what forms the balance of this chapter.

6.3 What might be

Before we reconsider how to compute and display summaries of blood sugar data let us first consider what are the key questions that these data may help to answer? By my estimation there are three questions:

(i) How am I doing overall? This is a long-term question that focuses on the blood sugar levels over extended periods of time to evaluate the efficacy of the various strategies being employed to control it.

(ii) How large are the variations in blood sugar level that take place over the course of the day due to normal daily events like eating meals, exercising, sleeping?

(iii) Are there any unusual excursions in blood sugar? How large are they? What causes them?

Each of these three questions has obvious medical implications. The first is the overall evaluation of the therapy. If the therapy has the character desired it means that whatever is being done is working. But if all we find is that the average blood sugar is too high, there are no immediate clues to aid in remediation.

The second question is primarily intermediate in character. We must know how much variation is usual before we can answer the third question, what is unusual? Management of blood sugar means more than keeping its typical amount in a particular range. It also is important to keep its variation within pre-specified bounds (e.g. between 80 and 140 mg/dl). The answer to this question can be both descriptive and prescriptive. If blood sugar shows unusually large variation before and after dinner, then one ought to consider eating less at dinner-time. Such a result is important and is unavailable solely from the answer to question one.

The third question is of least importance to the physician, but of potentially greatest import to the patient, for large excursions from what is normal will invariably have an associated story (e.g. a large cookie or an ice cream cone or too much beer and too many pretzels). Because each excursion has a specific story it also suggests an obvious remediation; don't do it any more. It is the immediate, clear and specific feedback from the answer to question (iii) that has the greatest likelihood of aiding the patient to shape his or her behavior and thus better control blood sugar.

In addition, as we will see, these are not independent questions. By estimating the pattern of daily variation, we should be able to obtain a more reliable estimate of long-term trends. Even a single isolated large excursion can have a significant effect on both the estimated daily variation and the long-term trend when these are represented by averages. I propose a simple method to address both of these problems with the result of providing better information to both doctor and patient.

What is the best way to answer these three questions and to convey those answers to the patient? The current approach is a listing of numbers—either the actual readings themselves, or three different averages (7, 14 and 30 day averages). Neither a list of numbers nor the use of averages is the best that we can do—and in combination they are worse still. My approach to summarization uses resistant statistical methods and my approach to presentation is graphical.

What is a resistant method? In short, it is a method that is not affected by a few unusual points. A median is resistant, a mean is not.

Why resistant? The current method of summarizing blood sugar results is taking averages. An average is fine for some things, but because it uses all of the information equally it has some weaknesses. The idea of a summary is that it essentially says, "This is typical of the data, most of them lie nearby." The arithmetic mean satisfies this heuristic when the data follow a bell shaped curve. But it does not follow it when there are even just a few very unusual points.

For example consider the following blood sugar readings:

90, 93, 95, 102, 210

The mean is 118. Thus the mean is not in the middle of the data nor is it near to any of the readings. In fact if we subtract the mean from each reading we get a vector of *residuals*:

−28, −25, −23, −16, 82

Using the mean as the summary statistic has had two unfortunate results here. First it located the middle where there were no scores nearby, and second, it distributed the mislocation among all of the observations. A better characterization would have told us that most of the scores were near 95, but one was very far away at 210. That latter piece is of critical importance, for it is by having that one outlying observation pointed out that the patient could then look for a cause. If a probable cause can be identified, the patient can modify his or her behavior in the hope of avoiding similar excursions in the future.

A much more resistant alternative to the mean is the median, 95. The residuals are then,

−5, −2, 0, 7, 115

leaving no doubt which observation is the extreme outlier.

6.4 Smoothing

When we have data arranged over time, it is often helpful to find a smooth trace through an otherwise scattered or choppy plot of the data. A smooth trace can show the overall pattern, free of the "noise" of point-to-point variation. And— often more important—it can provide a central summary from which to notice isolated exceptions to the overall pattern.

A smooth trace through a sequence of values serves much the same function as a summary of the middle of a single batch of values: it provides a central summary and facilitates identifying exceptions. And, for reasons that will be clear presently, smooth traces can suffer from the same sensitivity to isolated excursions as we saw with the mean.

One common way to find a smooth trace is to take local averages of values in the sequence. The result is called a *running mean* or sometimes a *moving average*. For example, Table 6.1 shows a sequence of blood sugar measurements and a running mean of 3 smooth of these measurements. The first smooth value, 110.7, is found as the mean of 104, 117 and 111.

But running means suffer from the same sensitivity to outlying values as we saw for means. Figure 6.2 shows a sequence of blood sugar measurements with a single outlying value (due to a glucose tolerance test), and the smooth found by running means of 3.

The data points are measured blood sugar levels. The connecting curve represents the smooth values. Note the boost in the curve that results from the contamination of the 3-smooth values by a single outlying value. If we used a larger smoothing window, say a running mean every five points instead of three, the excursion caused by the one outlying point would be smaller, but more points would be affected.

Because each smooth value averages three data values, the extreme value contaminates three of the values in the smooth trace. What may be of greater concern, the residuals—the difference between the data and the smooth—are also contaminated. It is the residuals that a patient would look at to be alerted to, a

TABLE 6.1 **A sequence of seven blood sugar measurements (mg/dl) and a running mean of three smooth of these measurements**

Blood sugar	Smooth
104	•
117	110.7
111	114.3
115	116.3
123	116.7
112	116.3
117	101.7

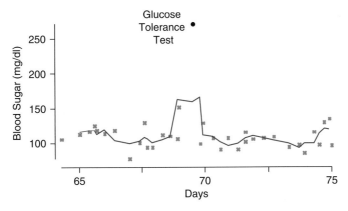

Figure 6.2 Thirty-seven data points taken over 10 days. The smooth connecting function is a running mean every three points.

deviation from the overall trend that might require attention. But, as Figure 6.3 shows, this approach could raise false alarms.

When looking at the residuals from a 3-smooth average of blood sugar levels, when one original value was unusually high (in this case, due to a glucose tolerance test), the residuals show the spike, but also suggest two blood sugar levels that only appear to be low because the spike has contaminated their smooth values.

The solution is to use a resistant smoothing method based on running medians instead. Resistant smoothers often give a less smooth trace, so special methods (beyond the scope of this chapter) can be used to improve the smoothness of the trace.

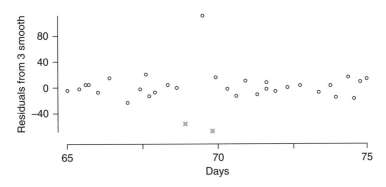

Figure 6.3 The residuals of the data points from the smooth curve shown in Figure 6.2.

6.5 An example

The subject is a 63-year-old male in generally good health. He is 6' 4" tall and weighed 230 pounds at the time of diagnosis. He exercises robustly five days a week, and has done so for his entire adult life.

Shown in Figure 6.4 is a plot of his fasting blood sugar taken over the past 15 years. From 1992 until 2005 it was under 140 mg/dl, but even in 2005 was trending upward portending a pre-diabetic condition.

In 2006 the annual result increased profoundly to 183 and the patient was told to lose 5 pounds and come back in 6 months. Six months later the patient returned 10 pounds lighter with fasting blood sugar of 249. He was diagnosed at that point as a type 2 diabetic and various corrective actions were taken. Specifically,

(i) A one-gram-a-day dosage of Metformin was prescribed and then titrated up to two grams a day over a two week period.

(ii) The patient limited his food intake to 2500 calories a day divided into 40% carbohydrates, 30% fats and 30% proteins, and the caloric intake was spread more evenly across the day.

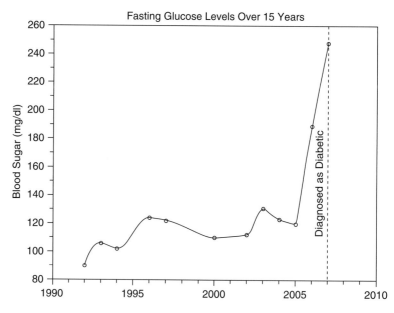

Figure 6.4 Fifteen years of fasting blood sugar tests showing both a pre-diabetic condition indicated by steady increases and the obvious onset of diabetes in 2006.

(iii) Exercise was increased from an hour a day to 90 minutes.

(iv) He was given a blood sugar sensing meter and began to check glucose levels 4–5 times a day.

The readings, taken using the device described earlier in this chapter, over a period two months are displayed in three plots. The first one, shown here as Figure 6.5, reflects all of the readings shown sequentially with a resistantly smoothed curve superimposed over them. It shows a steep decline of typical blood sugar as treatment began with a leveling off after the first month. We also note that the variation around the plotted curve continues to diminish beyond the initial month.

The decline in blood sugar has four plausible causes: medication, change in diet, change in exercise and the patient's loss of 25 more pounds. Because all of these things took place simultaneously we cannot partition the improvement in blood sugar levels among these four changes.

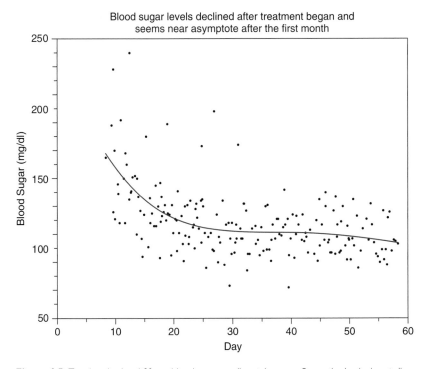

Figure 6.5 Two-hundred and fifteen blood sugar readings taken over 2 months, beginning at diagnosis. Superimposed over the readings is a curve indicating the outcome of the treatments being used to control blood sugar.

While we can see the variation across days, and roughly within each day, the within-day variation is more obvious if we make a plot that has the 24 hours of the day on the horizontal axis and the hourly *blood sugar effects* on the vertical. Blood sugar effects, in this instance, are what result after we subtract the resistant curve in Figure 6.5 from the actual blood sugar levels—thus what we plot has been adjusted for the long-term trend. We then aggregate across days and fit a resistant curve. Such a plot is shown as Figure 6.6.

The curve shown in Figure 6.6 indicates clearly that the typical range of variation over the course of a day is about 40 mg/dl. We see obvious spikes after each meal as well as a big drop when blood sugar is measured after noon-time exercise.

The third descriptive plot is of the residuals. This is a plot of blood sugar levels after removing the daily trend effects shown in Figure 6.5 and the daily effects shown in Figure 6.6. What remains are the unusual changes in blood sugar not accounted for by those other two effects. The residual plot is shown as Figure 6.7. One can easily see how it is the most immediately useful diagnostic plot for the patient. Each large residual should have a story associated with it. I have indicated just a few. We note that most large residuals occurred early

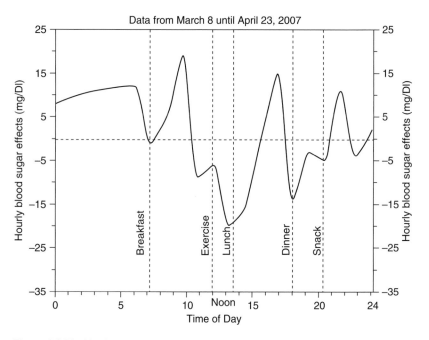

Figure 6.6 The blood sugar readings collapsed over days and summarized to show the typical daily variation. The plot is annotated to explain the variations.

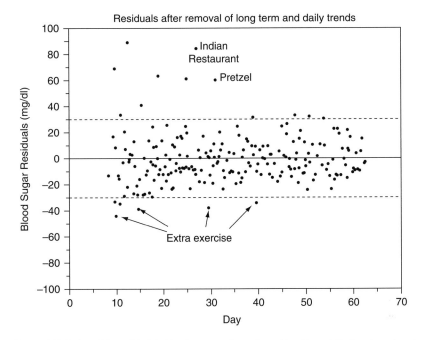

Figure 6.7 A plot of the residuals in blood sugar readings after subtracting out the long-term trend and the daily variation. Some unusual points are annotated to indicate probable cause.

in treatment before the patient's blood sugar had stabilized. The unusually low readings were invariably due to exercise. The two large positive residuals that occurred more than two weeks after diagnosis were due to specific eating events. This plot makes it clear that these are to be avoided in the future.

6.6 Conclusions

Diabetes is a dangerous disease that is spreading quickly. To be fully effective its treatment requires the full participation of the patient. Moreover it typically requires the patient to lose weight and exercise regularly, two things that are difficult to do for most people. It is my contention that by providing immediate and easily understood feedback on the relationship between the patient's diet and exercise on blood sugar it will help to reinforce proper behavior. I suggest that the use of average blood sugar has flaws that are easily ameliorated through the use of resistant methods such as the one I have described here. In addition, by providing the results in a graphic form the feedback is more vivid. Note that the word "graphic" in ordinary speech means "literal lifelikeness" but when used to describe an iconic visual display of data its meaning is almost exactly the opposite.

We see the same lesson we learned in Chapter 2, that a single display may not be sufficient to convey the richness of the data or answer the different questions that might be asked of them. I contend that by partitioning the blood sugar results into three pieces we highlight those aspects of the information that both clinician and patient need. Specifically, the overall trend curve illustrated in Figure 6.5 provides a clear and accurate summary of the efficacy of the treatment vis-à-vis blood sugar. At the same time the residual plot illustrated in Figure 6.7 allows the patient to see immediately the extent to which a specific action has affected blood sugar and hence implicitly suggests changes in future behavior. The explicit depiction of residuals from a resistant smooth makes clear how important is the accurate recording of the details of eating and exercise, for only through careful records can the stories of the residuals be told and acted upon.

Losing weight, and keeping it off, is universally acknowledged to be extraordinarily difficult. There are many reasons for this. One is that we have to eat so, unlike smoking, we cannot just quit eating. We have to eat less and avoid some foods. I contend that one reason for this being so hard to accomplish is that there is no immediate feedback. We can weigh ourselves in the morning, watch our diet carefully all day, and when we weigh ourselves again in the evening there is little or no discernable change. Similarly, we could eat like a pig all day and still see no short-term change. Blood sugar is very different. One misstep and it jumps skyward. Such immediate feedback, combined with the dire consequences of failure, makes adhering to a proper dietary regime easier (but by no means easy). The procedure I have outlined here provides an accurate estimate of unusual readings quickly.

Last, it seems sensible to discuss implementation of this approach. Of course this implementation is not device dependent. When there is an iPhone App to test blood sugar the same approach would apply. Nevertheless, the current blood meters are wondrous devices that already have in their innards the hardware necessary to implement this method. They have plenty of storage and, even if they didn't, adding more would be very cheap. Their screens can show statistical graphs as easily as they now show letters and other icons. To boost their capabilities in the way I suggest they want only some programming. Recent newspaper reports tell us that glucose meters will soon be blue-tooth enabled, so that they can instantly transmit results, via an iPhone, to our physician or other members of a diabetes support group. It isn't hard to imagine how such immediate information could be used.

CHAPTER 7

A second look at second opinions, with hip fractures as an example

7.1 Introduction

When faced with a serious medical decision we are often advised to get a second opinion[1]. This advice is in response to the reality that medical diagnoses, like all other human endeavors, vary. Getting multiple opinions helps us to determine what treatment pathway represents the consensus of medical wisdom. This advice is as wise in this region as diversifying one's portfolio is in the financial domain. It may not prevent catastrophe, but it is the safest way to bet.

But sometimes getting a second opinion is impossible, or at the very least impractical. Consider the following scenario:

Shirley, a 69-year-old female, caught her heel on a carpet and fell, hurting her hip. She was in severe pain, and was brought to a local hospital's emergency room. Her hip was X-rayed and it was quickly determined that she had fractured the neck of her left femur. There are two treatment options:

(i) The broken end of the bone can be removed and replaced with an artificial joint, or

(ii) The fracture can be treated with pins to align and stabilize the bone and promote fracture healing.

The first option represents major surgery with its attendant risks and a substantial recuperation time. The second option is performed through small slits in the skin and the risks and recuperation time is much less. Which procedure is appropriate depends on whether the blood supply to the femoral head has been disrupted by the fracture. If it has been, a hip replacement is required. If it has not, the joint may be safely pinned.

An orthopedic surgeon examined Shirley's X-ray and recommended a hip replacement. It is late at night, he is the only hip specialist in the hospital, and Shirley is immobile and in pain. Her opportunities for a second opinion are severely limited. What options does she have other than to nod her head weakly and go forward with the surgery?

Perhaps her decision could be aided if she knew something about the surgeon's propensities. Does he typically lean toward a conservative approach? In which case his diagnosis for replacement would take on greater credibility. Or is his specialty hip replacements, and sees the need for them around every corner? Or, more generally, how consistent are surgeons in making such diagnoses? Is this diagnosis an easy one in which there would be general agreement on a course of action?

7.2 Hip fractures and their severity

Hip fractures are common injuries; more than 250,000 annually are treated in the US alone. These fractures can be located in the shaft of the bone or in the neck of the bone connecting the shaft to the head of the femur. Femoral neck fractures vary in their severity. Robert S. Garden, a prominent British orthopedic surgeon, described a four part classification represented in the four panels of Figure 7.1: a partial crack through the neck (Panel A), a crack that fully extends across the femur but is impacted (Panel B), a complete crack and a slight displacement of the bone (Panel C), and a complete break with extensive displacement (Panel D). These four degrees of severity are classified by categories I, II, III and IV respectively.

When the break is displaced, the blood vessels that traverse the neck to nourish the head of the femur are more likely to be disrupted, markedly increasing the risk that the head will become necrotic. Hence the clinical treatment for fractures of type III and IV is a hip replacement. By contrast, if the fracture is not displaced, preservation of the blood supply can be assumed and thus the fracture can be treated with pins to align and stabilize the bone. The intuitive assumption that hip replacement is a more major and drastic surgery is correct.

Because the clinical consequences of the diagnosis are profoundly different depending on how the fracture is classified, it is natural to ask how accurately orthopedic surgeons make such diagnoses. Unfortunately, it is not practical to

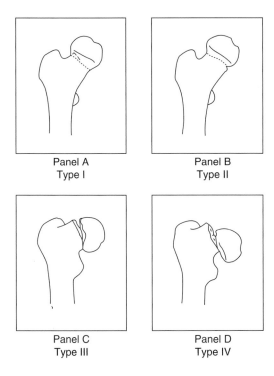

| Panel A | Panel B |
| Type I | Type II |

| Panel C | Panel D |
| Type III | Type IV |

answer the question of accuracy with reference to a "gold standard" because a patient's true condition is typically not observed directly: the surgical dissection and manipulation performed during hip replacement will displace even those fractures that were not displaced pre-operatively, whereas the pinning procedure is performed through 1 cm slits in the skin using X-ray guidance and not examined directly. Thus, *all* fractures that were pre-operatively diagnosed as displaced, correctly or otherwise, will be discovered to be displaced when examined under direct visualization in the operating room; and all fractures that were diagnosed as non-displaced will never be subject to direct visualization and independent confirmation.

7.3 How consistent are surgeons' judgments of hip fracture severity: The evidence

So far, while poor Shirley has been lying in bed suffering, we have been theorizing in advance of any facts. To aid her decision, Joseph Bernstein, an orthopedic surgeon at the University of Pennsylvania, gathered together X-rays of 15

TABLE 7.1 **The severity of 15 hip fractures classified by 12 orthopedic surgeons**

Physician	Case															Physician Mean	Effect
	1	2	3	4	5	6	7	8	9	10	11	12	13	14	15		
A	1	2	1	2	2	2	3	4	3	4	3	4	3	3	4	2.7	−0.4
B	1	2	1	1	2	4	3	2	4	3	4	3	4	4	4	2.8	−0.3
C	1	2	2	1	2	3	3	3	3	4	4	3	4	4	4	2.9	−0.3
D	1	1	2	1	2	4	3	3	4	4	3	4	4	4	4	2.9	−0.2
E	1	2	2	2	2	3	3	3	4	4	4	4	4	4	4	3.1	−0.1
F	2	1	2	3	3	2	4	4	2	4	4	4	4	4	4	3.1	0.0
G	2	1	2	1	3	3	4	3	4	4	4	4	4	4	4	3.1	0.0
H	1	2	2	3	2	4	3	4	3	3	4	4	4	4	4	3.1	0.0
I	2	2	2	1	3	3	4	4	4	4	4	4	4	4	4	3.3	0.1
J	1	3	2	4	2	4	4	4	4	4	4	4	4	4	4	3.5	0.3
K	1	2	3	4	4	4	4	4	4	4	4	4	4	4	4	3.6	0.5
L	2	2	3	3	4	4	4	4	4	4	4	4	4	4	4	3.6	0.5
Case Means	1.3	1.8	2.0	2.2	2.6	3.3	3.5	3.5	3.6	3.8	3.8	3.8	3.9	3.9	4.0	3.1	

different broken hips. He then convinced 12 eminent orthopedic surgeons to classify the fractures according to the Garden scheme just described. A slightly modified sample of the results he obtained are shown in Table 7.1.

The entries in the table are the Garden categories 1, 2, 3 and 4. The table is ringed with summaries that may need some explanation. At the bottom are case means, which summarize the judgments of all surgeons. Cases 1, 2, 3 and 4 were all judged, on average, to be good candidates for pinning. Cases 6 through 15 were all judged severe enough to require a hip replacement. Case 5 was equivocal and there was genuine disagreement among the surgeons. In this case getting even 12 opinions would not help in settling the issue. But let us focus on Case 3. On average it was judged a Garden 2, a prime candidate for pinning, yet if the patient's initial diagnosis came from either Surgeon K or Surgeon L, and there was no second opinion, there would be an artificial hip in her immediate future.

Now let us shift our attention to the next to last column on the right, labeled "Physician Mean." This column represents the average rating given out by each physician over all 15 cases. In a very real sense, this represents each physician's propensity toward doing a hip replacement. While there are differences among the physicians, they range from an average of 2.7 to 3.6, a difference from one extreme to the other of less than one Garden category. The average over all physicians and over all cases is 3.1, indicating that this selection of cases represents a sample of relatively severe injuries. The very last column, labeled "Physician Effect" is obtained by simply subtracting the overall mean, 3.1, from each physician's average. The effect represents how far each physician's judgments are from the group mean. So physicians A through E are somewhat more likely to recommend pinning than average, and physicians I through L somewhat less likely to. Note that the average effect, by construction, must be zero.

The physician effects are very important, for we can use them to adjust each physician's judgments to undo their propensity toward one extreme or the other. Such an adjustment is very easy, we simply subtract each physician's effect from all of their judgments. The adjusted classifications are shown in Table 7.2.

TABLE 7.2 The severity of 15 hip fractures classified by 12 orthopedic surgeons: Adjusted by surgeon propensity

Physician	Case															Physician
	1	2	3	4	5	6	7	8	9	10	11	12	13	14	15	Mean
A	1.4	2.4	1.4	2.4	2.4	2.4	3.4	4.4	3.4	4.4	3.4	4.4	3.4	3.4	4.4	3.1
B	1.3	2.3	1.3	1.3	2.3	4.3	3.3	2.3	4.3	3.3	4.3	3.3	4.3	4.3	4.3	3.1
C	1.3	2.3	2.3	1.3	2.3	3.3	3.3	3.3	3.3	4.3	4.3	3.3	4.3	4.3	4.3	3.1
D	1.2	1.2	2.2	1.2	2.2	4.2	3.2	3.2	4.2	4.2	3.2	4.2	4.2	4.2	4.2	3.1
E	1.1	2.1	2.1	2.1	2.1	3.1	3.1	3.1	4.1	4.1	4.1	4.1	4.1	4.1	4.1	3.1
F	2.0	1.0	2.0	3.0	3.0	2.0	4.0	4.0	2.0	4.0	4.0	4.0	4.0	4.0	4.0	3.1
G	2.0	1.0	2.0	1.0	3.0	3.0	4.0	3.0	4.0	4.0	4.0	4.0	4.0	4.0	4.0	3.1
H	1.0	2.0	2.0	3.0	2.0	4.0	3.0	4.0	3.0	3.0	4.0	4.0	4.0	4.0	4.0	3.1
I	1.9	1.9	1.9	0.9	2.9	2.9	3.9	3.9	3.9	3.9	3.9	3.9	3.9	3.9	3.9	3.1
J	0.7	2.7	1.7	3.7	1.7	3.7	3.7	3.7	3.7	3.7	3.7	3.7	3.7	3.7	3.7	3.1
K	0.5	1.5	2.5	3.5	3.5	3.5	3.5	3.5	3.5	3.5	3.5	3.5	3.5	3.5	3.5	3.1
L	1.5	1.5	2.5	2.5	3.5	3.5	3.5	3.5	3.5	3.5	3.5	3.5	3.5	3.5	3.5	3.1
Case Means	1.3	1.8	2.0	2.2	2.6	3.3	3.5	3.5	3.6	3.8	3.8	3.8	3.9	3.9	4.0	3.1

There are several aspects of this table that are of note. First, the average rating of each case remains the same. This is a consequence of the average effect being zero. Second, the mean rating for each physician is now, by construction, the same, 3.1, and so the differential effect of being diagnosed by any particular physician is zero. Last, and most important to poor Shirley, let us look at the adjusted ratings for Case 3 by physicians K and L. Before adjustment they were both 3, indicating a hip replacement. After adjustment, they are the more equivocal 2.5, indicating a profound uncertainty regarding treatment. With a rating like this there is evidence to justify enduring the delay and discomfort associated with getting another opinion. And, in this case, the second opinion would likely tilt the diagnosis toward the gentler option.

7.4 Where can this go from here?

A second medical opinion, defined traditionally, means asking another physician for guidance in diagnosis and treatment. In the situation of an emergency room and a broken hip, getting a traditional second opinion may be so difficult that unless there is a clear justification for the substantial extra effort, the only strategy seemed to be to trust in the initial surgeon's judgment. But if we redefine what we mean by a second opinion, in this case getting opinions from the same physician on previous cases, we can gather evidence that can usefully be brought to bear. It isn't hard to imagine that once medical records are computerized one could easily have access to each physician's tendencies and be able to make the sort of adjustment I used here.

We can speculate that once such information is available to physicians themselves, they will adjust their own judgments to bring them closer to the expert consensus. Similarly, if outcome measures are also available (e.g. if many marginal cases that were pinned eventually failed because the head of the femur became necrotic, indicating that the blood supply was, in fact, compromised) physicians might adjust their judgments upward. To accomplish this requires just two things: evidence and the willingness to act on it.

CHAPTER 8

False positives or is a pound of prevention worth an ounce of cure

8.1 Introduction

In any detection problem, whether it is the early detection of disease or the detection of criminals or terrorists, there are two kinds of errors we can make. The first kind of error is when the test comes up negative incorrectly: where the person has the disease and we missed it. This is called a false negative. The second kind of error is when the test comes up positive incorrectly: when we prosecute an innocent person or detect a disease in a healthy person. This is called a false positive. Whenever what we are searching for is relatively rare, a terrorist in the United States or a cancerous tumor in the general population, the number of false positives can swamp the number of true positives. This phenomenon, though obvious once we get used to it, is not given the attention it deserves in most public discussions. This is unfortunate for, as we shall see, false positives often have an unexpectedly profound effect on the efficacy of any detection strategy[1].

8.2 Example 1. Using mammograms for the early detection of breast cancer among women

Annually there are about 180,000 new cases of invasive breast cancer diagnosed in women in the US. About 40,000 of these women are expected to die from breast cancer. Breast cancer is second only to skin cancer as the most commonly diagnosed cancer, and second only to lung cancer in death rates. Among US. women. about 1 in 4 cancers are breast cancer and one in every eight US women can expect to be diagnosed with breast cancer at some time in their lives.

However some progress in the battle against the horrors of breast cancer has been made. Death rates have been declining over the last 20 years due to a combination of early detection and improved treatment. The first steps in early detection are self-examination and mammograms. The strategy is then to investigate any unusual lumps found with these relatively benign procedures by using more invasive, yet revealing methods—most particularly a biopsy.

How effective are mammograms? One measure of their effectiveness is characterized in a simple statistic. If a mammogram is found to be positive, what is the probability that it is cancer? We can estimate this probability from a fraction that has two parts. The numerator is the actual number of breast cancers found and the denominator is the number of positive mammograms. The denominator contains both the true and the false positives.

The numerator first: it is 180,000 cases.

The denominator has two parts: the true positives, 180,000, plus the false positives. How many of these are there? Each year there are 33.5 million mammograms given in the US. The accuracy of mammograms varies from 80% to 90% depending on circumstances[2]. For the purposes of this discussion let's assume the more accurate figure of 90% accuracy. What this means is that when there is a cancer, 90% of the time it will be found, and when there is no cancer 90% of the time it will indicate no cancer. But this means that 10% of the time it will indicate a possible cancer when there is none. So, 10% of 33.5 million mammograms yield 3.35 million false positives. Thus the denominator of our fraction is 180,000 plus 3.35 million, or roughly 3.5 million positive mammograms.

Therefore the probability of someone with a positive mammogram having breast cancer is:

$$180,000/3.5 \text{ million or about } 5\%. \tag{8.1}$$

That means that 95% of the women who receive the horrible news that the mammogram has revealed something suspicious, and that they must return for further testing, possibly including a biopsy, are just fine.

Is a test with this level of accuracy worth doing? Let us consider first the costs of doing the test and then some alternatives.

First the cost in terms of money. In the US mammograms cost between $100 and $200 each. Let's use the cheaper figure. So for 33.5 million mammograms the cost (conservatively) is $3.35 billion. Next, the cost of a biopsy varies between about $1,000 for a thin needle aspiration and $5,000 for a fuller surgical procedure. Let's use the lower number. So to biopsy the 3.5 million positive mammograms the cost would be at least $3.5 billion. So far the cost is just shy of $7 billion.

Now let's add on some other costs. Mammograms take at least 2–3 hours out of a working day, and biopsies at least 4 hours, often more. So, figuring conservatively, the two tests use up 70 million and 14 million hours, respectively, of women's time. 84 million hours at even just $15/hour is an opportunity cost of $1.2 billion.

And last, how can we measure the emotional cost of the anxiety between the time one is told that there is an abnormality seen in the mammogram and the all-clear from the biopsy? We might also add in the false positives from biopsies and the complications that sometimes ensue after a biopsy (e.g. a staph infection). I will not try to place a dollar value on this aspect, but by any measure it is not a cost to be ignored when trying to value a mammogram.

We have a conservative estimate of the annual US costs of mammograms: $8 billion. In return for this cost we have the earlier detection of 180,000 breast cancers (actually 162,000, since 10% of the 180,000 that are eventually uncovered were missed in the initial mammogram). By dividing the costs of testing by the total number uncovered we can estimate the average cost of initial diagnosis, or

$$\$8\,\text{billion}/162,000 = \$49,000. \tag{8.2}$$

Thus it costs at least $49,000 to diagnose one case of breast cancer. And, for the unfortunate victims of the disease, this is only the start of the costs of treatment.

But this is the cost of detection. It is surely more relevant to weigh the costs of detection against the likelihood of extending the patient's life. Here the picture gets more complicated. In 2009 Nielson Gotzsche conducted a rigorous review of dozens of high quality studies of the value of mammography, encompassing more than a half-million women. He concluded,

EXAMPLE 1. USING MAMMOGRAMS | 107

. . . for every 2,000 women invited for screening throughout the ten years, one will have her life prolonged. In addition, 10 healthy women, who would not have been diagnosed if there had not been screening, will be diagnosed as breast cancer patients and will be treated unnecessarily. It is thus not clear whether screening does more good than harm.

Both aspects of this remarkable conclusion deserve our attention. First, that only one out of every 2,000 women screened will have her life extended. In the US, where 33.5 million women are annually screened, this means that 16,700 will have their lives extended because of the treatment triggered by the early detection afforded by a mammogram.

This provides a new metric for our calculation of the value of a mammogram. Suppose we narrow the question we asked to, "what is the detection cost for each life that is extended by that early detection?"

To calculate this we merely divide the total cost of screenings ($8 billion) in the US by the number of women whose lives were extended (16,700) yielding

$$\$8\,\text{billion}/16{,}700 = \$479{,}000. \tag{8.3}$$

A very large amount indeed, and it does not include any of the costs of treatment, nor the associated emotional costs[3]. It also does not include the costs of both lives and treasure associated with Gotzsche's ominous second conclusion, that ten healthy women per 2,000 will be treated unnecessarily and hence suffer the inevitable injury that modern cancer treatment entails. What sort of unnecessary treatment will they be subjected to? Is it just the relatively benign biopsy? Or is it something more? Gotzsche expands,

Finally, carcinoma in situ is much more likely to be detected with mammography and it is known that although less than half of the cases will progress to be invasive (Nielsen, 1987), these women will nevertheless be treated with surgery, drugs, and radiotherapy.

I have not tried to calculate the shortening of lives of the 167,000 healthy women who were incorrectly treated for breast cancer, but such a calculation would be crucial to balance the value of early screening.

Can we do anything to shift the balance? Yes, we must reduce the size of the denominator. But so long as the ratio of healthy to sick people is so large, improving the accuracy of the test yields only limited help (going from 90% accurate to say 95% doesn't put much of a dent in it). The only real help would be reducing the number of mammograms administered that have only a tiny chance of revealing anything. Perhaps only women with a family history as well as those over 50, or maybe over 60.

More light was shed on this very difficult triage decision in a September 2010 report on the results of a Norwegian study of the efficacy of mammograms, published in the *New England Journal of Medicine*. This is the first study that examined the value of the early detection possible through mammograms when coupled with modern treatments such as hormonal therapy and other targeted drugs. In it the researchers compared the breast cancer death rates for women who had early detection with mammograms to those whose cancer was detected later after the tumor had grown enough to be noticed manually. They found that the difference in survival rates were small enough to be chalked up to chance.

The Norwegian result lends support to the growing concern over the widespread use of mammograms, without regard to the often profoundly negative consequences for the many women who were on the receiving end of a false positive diagnosis. The price of false positives was worthwhile when successful treatment was dependent on early detection. But now modern treatments have seemingly thrown the earlier practice into a cocked hat.

My point is that these kinds of calculations emphasize that a screening device like a mammogram is not an unalloyed good. We must search for a balance to shape policy. I did not do the rough financial analysis in an attempt to try to weigh the value of a human life saved against some number of dollars. This is a difficult calculus for the money that is spent on unnecessary mammograms cannot be spent on other things that might have a greater positive impact on national health. No, my purpose was to suggest how hard it is to sharply limit a procedure that currently generates (in the US alone) more than 4 billion dollars a year for its practitioners.

I note without further comment the reactions to the Norwegian study from three physicians whose commitment to the continued use of mammograms varies[4]:

Dr. Barnett Kramer, associate director for disease prevention at the US National Institutes of Health. "This new study is very credible."

Dr. Carol Lee, a radiologist at Memorial Sloan-Kettering Cancer Center and chair of the breast imaging commission of the American College of Radiology, said that the new study "affirmed that mammography saves lives."

Dr. Laura Esserman, a professor of surgery and radiology at the University of California in San Francisco, said that it tells her "if you get the same treatment and the outcome is the same if you find the tumor earlier or later, then you don't make a difference when you find it early."

EXAMPLE 1. USING MAMMOGRAMS | 109

8.3 Example 2. Using the PSA (prostate-specific antigen) test for the early detection of prostate cancer among men

If the use of a detection technique as well known and long researched as a mammogram is problematic, how useful is a PSA test likely to be? Prostate cancer is one of the most common cancers. Current estimates are that this year in the US more than 185,000 men will be diagnosed with prostate cancer, and more than 29,000 men will die from the disease. The reason that the number who will die from it is only 16% of the number who are diagnosed has to do with when it is first detected and treated. The Prostate Cancer Foundation states that, "because approximately 90% of all prostate cancers are detected in the local and regional stages, the cure rate for prostate cancer is very high—nearly 100% of men diagnosed at this stage will be disease-free after five years."

This appears to be a powerful argument for universal screening, although all of the authoritative sources waffle about such a recommendation. The American Cancer Society recommends that "health care professionals should discuss the potential benefits and limitations of prostate cancer early detection testing with men before any testing begins. This discussion should include an offer for testing with the prostate specific antigen (PSA) blood test and digital rectal exam (DRE) yearly, beginning at age 50, to men who are at average risk of prostate cancer and have at least a 10-year life expectancy."

They say "offered," but do they mean that they recommend it? How well qualified is a typical patient to make this kind of decision? One would think that after such a discussion most patients would say to their physician, "what do you think I should do?"

Reading a little further we find the recommendation, "If, after this discussion, a man asks his health care professional to make the decision for him, he should be tested."

So the idea, stated syllogistically, is:

Major Premise: Prostate cancer is common and deadly, but detected early is almost 100% curable.

Minor Premise: It can be detected with a PSA test, which is cheap, easy and painless.

Inevitable conclusion by the patient: Please include the PSA test as part of my annual check-up.

Now let us go a little more slowly and see what the consequences of such a chain of reasoning.

First how many US men fall into the category of being "at-risk" (i.e. are over 50)? In round numbers there are about 46 million.

Suppose they are all tested. Again, a natural question is "If I am tested and found to have an elevated PSA, what are the chances that I have prostate cancer?"

Such a probability is a fraction that has, in its numerator, the number of actual cancers detected—185,000.

Its denominator has the total number of elevated PSAs, those generated by cancer and those positive PSAs that turn out to be false alarms. How many are there? Most men with an elevated PSA test result turn out not to have cancer; only 25% to 35% of men who have a biopsy due to an elevated PSA level actually have prostate cancer[5]. Let us use the larger number, 35%. That means that of about 530,000 men with an elevated PSA, 35% or 185,000 had cancer. What proportion of the men tested had an elevated PSA? That's hard to say, since what is considered elevated varies by age, by race and by prior condition, but a reasonable estimate is that the top 10% had an elevated PSA. That would mean that there must have been about 5.3 million PSA tests administered to have yielded 530,000 elevated ones, which in turn yielded 185,000 cancers.

Suppose we had a sudden spate of responsibility among American men over 50 and all 46 million of us ran out and had PSA tests. That would yield 4.6 million elevated tests requiring a biopsy to check. So the probability that we have prostate cancer, given that we had an elevated PSA is:

$$185,000/4,600,000 = 4\%. \qquad (8.4)$$

Is any test with an accuracy of only 4% worth doing? That would depend on the value of detecting the cancer versus the costs of not detecting it. The arguments about the efficacy of prostate cancer treatment are as much medical as they are statistical and must weigh the costs of the inevitable side effects against the anticipated increase in life expectancy, and we need not get into that. Instead let us just look at the costs of testing. The PSA test itself is cheap and easy, just one of many blood tests that can be done as part of a normal medical check-up. But what happens if all men over 50 in the US have a PSA? We would find that 4.6 million of us have an elevated value requiring a biopsy to adjudicate. The cheapest kind of biopsy is a "thin needle aspiration" and costs about $1,200. And it is not as easily accomplished as a blood test. So now we are adding $5.52 billion ($1,200 × 4.6 million) to the health tab. In addition to this cost are the opportunity costs associated with 4.6 million of us missing a day's work and hanging out at a hospital for something that is likely to take all day. And so, if

EXAMPLE 2. USING THE PSA TEST | 111

we divide the total cost of the test by the number of cancers detected we arrive at a figure somewhere well north of $30,000 to detect one prostate cancer. And we haven't begun to estimate the cost of lengthening one life, for the marginal value of treatment for prostate cancer over doing nothing is still being decided.[6]

Is this worth it? I don't know, since an answer to this depends on many things—the age of the patient, the prognosis, etc. But, and this is my main point, we should know this number before making any policy recommendations. Medical care is full of triage decisions. Money spent on one thing isn't available for another. $5.52 billion dollars spent on inoculations for children is likely to yield more fruit. But this too is a policy decision that must be armed with evidence. But evidence is too often countered with tales of genuine tragedy about how someone's life was lost, or saved, through early detection.

The plural of anecdote is not data.

8.4 Example 3. Using wiretaps to find terrorists[7]

The Federal Bureau of Investigation has incorrectly kept nearly 24,000 people on a terrorist watch list . . . while missing people with genuine ties to terrorism who should have been on the list.

The New York Times (May 7, 2009, p. A22)

As seen in the news report quoted above, false positives bedevil more than medical tests. Let us consider the very difficult problem faced by the Bush administration post-9/11. They felt that the safety of the nation was compromised and that all stops should be pulled out in the detection and arrest of terrorists in the United States. As part of their initiative they authorized a program of wiretaps and surveillance coupled with imprisonment. Ignoring the constitutional issues of warrantless wiretaps and imprisonment without trial, which have been debated for a long time, it seems worthwhile to try to get a sense of how successful such a program could be.

Let's assume that they were able to couple a program that wiretapped all phone calls received or placed in the United States with wonderful software that could tell within a half-dozen words whether a person was a terrorist or not with 99% accuracy. They would then forward the names of those so identified to the FBI for immediate action. Of course software of such accuracy doesn't exist, not even close, but let us for the moment assume it does and see where it takes us.

Let us further assume that there were 3,000 terrorists in hiding in the US. I don't mean ordinary murderers or thugs, but genuine terrorists whose goal is the spreading of terror and mayhem within the US. I don't know if 3,000 is the right number. It might be too large by a factor of ten, or too small by the same amount—but we can probably agree that the correct number is somewhere between 300 and 30,000. It is easy to repeat the following calculations for these bounds and confirm that our conclusions will not materially change. So let's stay with 3,000.

So now we ask, if you are identified as a terrorist, what is the probability that you are one?

As before, the estimate of this probability is a fraction that has the number of true terrorists in the numerator and the number of people identified as terrorists in the denominator—the true positives plus the false positives.

The numerator is 99% × 3,000 = 2,970.

The denominator is 2,970 plus 1% × 300 million = 3,002,970.

The second term in the denominator comes from listening in on everyone in the US, all 300 million of us and, since the identification software is 99% accurate, it makes a mistake 1% of the time. 1% of 300 million is 3 million.

For ease of calculation let's round the probability to

$$3,000/3,000,000 = 1/1,000,$$

or, in prose, if you are identified as a terrorist the chances are one in a thousand that you are one. This means that for every true terrorist shunted off to Guantanamo Bay, Cuba there are 999 innocent and, justifiably, angry citizens.

At this point we can easily experiment with alternative assumptions. If there are only 300 true terrorists the odds change to one in ten-thousand. If there are 30,000 true terrorists the odds become one in a hundred.

If the accuracy of the detection process is improved to 99.9% accurate, the odds become one in a hundred. If the detection process is 90% accurate the odds become one in ten-thousand. And so on.

This little experiment teaches us two important lessons:

First, it tells us that the sort of strategy examined here is unlikely to work and, further, when we hear a news report that a suspected terrorist hideout was bombed, and that 30 were killed, we should view the result with some skepticism, for it is not far-fetched to believe that most, if not all, of them were innocent. And the news report that began this section, telling of 24,000 false positives, should come as no surprise.

EXAMPLE 3. USING WIRETAPS TO FIND TERRORISTS | 113

> Second, this is a strategy for estimating the outcomes of various policies. We can make some broad assumptions about the true situations, even when we have only a vague knowledge of the truth. Then we can try out various alternative possibilities that span the range of credibility. If we find that even under the most optimistic of circumstances a particular policy can't work, we can dismiss it and consider others.

How can we develop a more workable policy to detect terrorists? Clearly we need to shrink the denominator. But how? Making the detection system more accurate than 99.9% is not likely. Indeed, even 99% accuracy is almost surely a pipedream. So the only thing left is to target who is wiretapped more tightly. We can all agree that we can probably exclude Danish grandmothers from our purview without loss of accuracy. As well as other, larger groups. But what this means is that we are using some sort of profiling—which has in it its own threats to civil liberties. And so a triage decision has to be made about the balance between general safety and equality under the law. A difficult discussion surely, but one that can be more informed through analyses like the one I have outlined here.

8.5 Example 4. Detecting criminals: Estimating the number of innocents in prison

As recently as the 1980s, it was extraordinarily rare for convicted prisoners to establish their innocence conclusively enough to get public attention. That changed with breakthroughs in DNA science. In the eighteen years between 1989 and 2007 there were more than 200 exonerations, including 15 who were sentenced to death, based on post-conviction DNA testing.

But it is Pollyannaish to believe that the DNA exonerations capture all of the imprisoned innocents. Quite the opposite, it is evidence that suggests that there are likely many thousands of other wrongly convicted people in prisons and jails around the country. And conversely, there are likely large numbers of guilty people still at large.

We can get a handle on the problem through the use of the same sort of educated guesswork we used in estimating the value of wholesale wiretaps to find terrorists.[8]

How many criminals are there in the US? Not just any criminals, but only those whose crimes justify imprisonment. I don't know how many in any given year. Probably well more than a thousand, but perhaps fewer than a million. To start let's pick a million as the number of annual criminals lurking out there. Next, let us assume that we are all equal before the law. By this I mean that when a crime is committed everyone is a suspect, although vast numbers of us will be eliminated from consideration very quickly. And last, let us say that the criminal justice system is 99% accurate. I'll define the "criminal justice system" as the sequence that includes detection, arrest, prosecution and punishment. This means that when a crime is committed 99% of the time the right person is found, tried, convicted and punished. And, in parallel, only 1% of the time is it the wrong person. I don't know what the right figure is for accuracy, but 99% seems high enough to not unfairly malign the criminal justice system. If you disagree with any of these numbers substitute in ones that you find more likely.

So we return the same question again—if you are imprisoned what are the chances that you are guilty?

The numerator is the number of guilty people convicted, which is 99% of a million, or 990,000.

The denominator has these 990,000 plus 1% of the 300,000,000 of the rest of the US, or 3 million.

Doing the arithmetic we have

$$990,000/(3,990,000) = 25\%, \tag{8.5}$$

or, with these assumptions, 75% of the people annually sentenced to prison are innocent.

Of course these assumptions are surely wrong. The probability of a false positive is probably much lower than the probability of a false negative, for our legal system has long ago realized that it is almost always better to free a guilty person than to imprison an innocent one. In addition, if here are one million crimes there will not be 4 million people imprisoned. But this initial version conveys the idea that even with remarkable accuracy we should not be surprised to find a very large proportion of innocent people in prison.

A different model that is more realistic but gives essentially the same results might be a two stage process in which a pool of suspects are collected. This pool contains 99% of the guilty ones (990,000 again) and only 1% of innocent ones (3,000,000). Then the second stage selects 1 million people from this pool, each with equal likelihood, to go to prison. This would yield the proportion of guilty people in prison shown in equation 8.5.

EXAMPLE 4. DETECTING CRIMINALS | 115

8.6 Tidying up

Some ideas only sound good if you say them fast. In this chapter we discussed four somewhat disparate schemes for detection, each of which may sound good when you first hear it, but the prospective value of all of them rapidly diminish once we look more carefully. They all share the same issue, an overwhelming number of false positives, and so by the time we reached the fourth one I am sure you were far ahead of me in recognizing it. The key issue underlying all four situations is measuring the cost of prevention. Mixed in with this issue is a more subtle and difficult one relating to a small cost spread over many compared with a dear cost for very few.

My contention is that thoughtful consideration of policy for each these four strategies should be based on their supporting facts and not on the passion with which they are held by their supporters.

CHAPTER 9

Assessing long-term risk with shorter-term data

9.1 Introduction[1]

In the October 16, 2010 issue of *The New York Times*, science reporter Gina Kolata published an article about two classes of drugs[2] whose risk changes after long-term use. As she explains, "The difficulty is in figuring out how to assess the safety of drugs that will be taken for decades, when the clinical trials last at most a few years."

How indeed? One solution might be to insist that drug usage be limited only to the length of time supported by both animal trials and human clinical trials. But requiring long-term clinical trials before approval is likely to make long-term usage of a drug prohibitively expensive. It would also effectively postpone the use of possibly useful drugs longer than seems reasonable. Are there other options?

The beginnings of a solution would be to institute continuous data-gathering for all drugs with an associated on-going data analysis, much like what is done in statistical process control. There may also need to be some sort of limitation on liability if a problem arises in long-term use that could not have been foreseen with short-term data (e.g. the increases in heart risk that were discovered in those who used Vioxx long-term for the treatment of arthritis). This is precisely what current practice is in the US, for after drugs receive final Food and Drug Administration (FDA) approval and are put into use for the general population, a Phase IV "post-approval" clinical trial is said to commence (or what is called a "post-marketing surveillance trial"). Safety surveillance is intended to detect rare or long-term adverse effects or unintended consequences over the larger patient base now using the drug. Adverse effects identified in these Phase IV trials can result in drugs being recalled or restricted for certain uses.

For example, one of the drugs of concern in Kolata's article, Avandia, has been monitored regularly. On November 14, 2007, the FDA added the warning that patients with underlying heart disease or at high risk of heart attack may be at increased risk for heart failure or heart attack. And in September of 2010, after more long-term usage data had accumulated, FDA regulators in the United States and their European counterparts simultaneously introduced restrictions ensuring that Avandia would no longer be widely available.

Prescription drugs withdrawn because of Phase IV trials capture major media attention as well as substantial legal interest (e.g. in individual and class-action lawsuits). Some of the names of discontinued drugs are familiar: Ephedra, Fen-phen, Vioxx, Thalidomide, DES, Baycol, among many others.

This monitoring is, of course, a matter of national interest, and must be independent of the pharmaceutical industry producing the drugs in the first place. At present, pharmaceutical companies pay a fee to the FDA for approval of a new medical procedure or drug. After approval, Phase IV trials could also be funded in the same way, possibly as a function of sales and profits, and through an agency separate from and not unduly influenced by the pharmaceutical industry.

But can the practice of modern statistics and careful experimental design provide additional help to allow a peek into the distant future derived from information gathered in the here-and-now? The answer is yes, and some suggestions as to how this might be done are presented in the remainder of this chapter.

9.2 Method I. Low-dose extrapolation

In so-called Delaney Clause research, a technique has evolved to determine the carcinogenic effect of food additives. We often read reports of such research in the popular media, but it is usually so poorly explained that most readers scoff at its outcomes. A typical report of, say, an artificial sweetener, might tell us of a small carcinogenic effect found in experimental animals when they received a dosage equivalent to the amount ingested in 20 cases of diet drinks a day. Such a report is summarily discounted—we recognize that the dosage is absurd and that anyone who thinks that such an experiment has any bearing on real-life must be either demented or a fool. Truth be told, this inference may not be fully justified. The problem researchers face is that if they used normal dosages, the life expectancy of the experimental animals might not be long enough for the effect to manifest itself.[3] Or, even if it were, the probability of cancer might be so small that the experiment would require an impractically large number of animals. So, instead, they divide up the animals into several treatment groups. One might get the equivalent of 20 cases of diet soda a day, a second might get 10 cases, a third 5, a fourth just one case, and the last group, the control group, would get no artificial sweetener. In each group, the proportion of animals developing a tumor is recorded.

Now imagine a graph, very much like the hypothetical one shown as Figure 9.1, in which the horizontal axis has the amount of sweetener ingested each day, and the vertical axis the probability of developing a tumor. If this probability increases with dosage level (as for sweetener B), it is straightforward to fit a curve to these data points and extrapolate down to the region of what might be considered normal dosages. This provides an estimate of the carcinogenic effect of this artificial sweetener.[4] Note that if there is no trend with dosage (as for

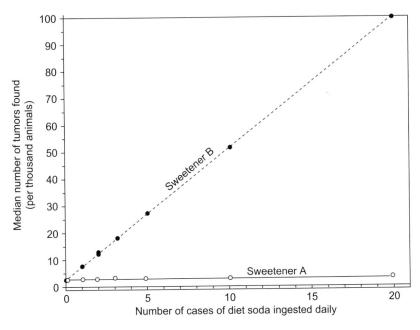

Figure 9.1 Hypothetically low-dose extrapolation curves for two artificial sweeteners.

sweetener A), and the incidence of tumors were no different for the experimental groups than for the control group, we have experimental evidence that the sweetener has no carcinogenic effect.

The next step, which has plenty of its own perils, involves extrapolating from laboratory animals to humans—often a very big step indeed. Obviously, such extrapolations are always tricky, but this is a practical approach to what is a vexing problem.

A modification of this approach might help us to estimate the long-term effects of a drug. One variation could keep track of side effects as a function of length of usage, and extrapolate outward to the long term. If effects are subtle, they may be unseen for those time periods suitable for pre-approval testing. This might be helped by simultaneously boosting dosages in experimental animals (not in human clinical trials), hoping to accelerate the side effects and the estimation of long-term effects. This approach is akin to what is reviewed next.

9.3 Method 2. Accelerated life testing

In the local hardware store are "long-life" light bulbs for sale with a life expectancy of 50,000 hours printed on their packaging. Because 50,000 hours is 5.7 years of continuous burning, an obvious question to ask is: "How can they know this?" Of course, they might have developed this new bulb and set a collection of them together in a long rack, turned them on and waited until half had died. But how could any research and development team's value be assessed if it took almost 6 years for management to find out if what they said was correct? And how could a manufacturer of bulbs keep a competitive edge if they had such a long delay in getting their new products to market? Clearly, that is not what they are likely to do. Instead, failure is accelerated under special conditions to estimate what would happen under normal operating conditions. For example, one set of bulbs engineered to operate properly at 110 volts—the US standard, might burn at 200 volts (they would, no doubt, die out relatively quickly), a second set at 190 volts, a third at 180, and so on. After noting the median length of time to failure for the bulbs in each group, they could make a graph of voltage by survival time and extrapolate down to 110 volts. Because it does involve extrapolation and an assumption that the effects of aging are akin to the effects of increased voltage, it is not a perfect solution, but it does provide a plausible answer.

Last week, in an ad for LED bulbs, the store claimed that these would be the last bulbs you need ever buy, for they would likely last longer than you would.

Obviously they made this claim for longevity without doing the standard experiment. They must have used some sort of accelerated life testing (or made the claim based upon experience with LEDs and a bit of blind faith).[5]

Another kind of accelerated life testing subjects a particular device to the kinds of wear-and-tear expected over a long period of time, but in a much shorter period. For example, in testing the robustness of car door hinges, a machine could open and close the door every five seconds, and continuously for several days. In that time the door has been operated the same number of times as might accumulate in ten years of normal use. Is this the same as normal use? Well no, because there are not the temperature changes, the rain, snow, wind, and the general aging of metal that can happen over a multi-year period. But it does provide some information. Coupled with a continuous monitoring of the car doors or other mechanical parts in real-life (a version of Phase IV trials for automobiles), this information can help revise longevity estimates as new data become available, and possibly trigger recalls (in 2011, think Toyota).

9.4 Conclusion

The parallels should be clear between the areas of application for accelerated life testing, and low-dose extrapolation, and the need to estimate the long-term side effects of drug treatments. We cannot know long-term effects from short-term data, but we can get plausible estimates through careful experimentation. These experiments make predictions about both long- and intermediate-term results. These extrapolations can be tested as data come in from collection in the field (Phase IV trials), and either confirm the inferences made that the drug treatment is safe, or, if disconfirming, allow immediate change of practice. These approaches are not perfect, but represent a practical solution to an important, but difficult, problem.

CHAPTER 10

A remarkable horse: An inquiry into the accuracy of medical predictions

A horse that can count to ten is a remarkable horse, it is not a remarkable mathematician.

Samuel Johnson

10.1 Introduction

A psychiatrist who knows a little statistics may be a remarkable psychiatrist, but he or she is not a remarkable statistician. Hence it is not remarkable that when we look at statistical reasoning applied by psychiatrists we find mysteries[1,2]. One such mystery, which is especially dramatic, manifests itself in the expert testimony surrounding the court case Barefoot v. Estelle (decided by the US Supreme Court on July 6, 1983). We shall use it to illustrate the problem. What follows is a lightly edited version of *an Amicus Curiae*[3] brief prepared by the American Psychiatric Association.

Petitioner Thomas A. Barefoot stood convicted by a Texas state court on August 7, 1978 for the murder of a police officer – one of five categories of homicides for which Texas law authorizes the imposition of the death penalty. Under capital sentencing procedures established after the Texas Court's decision in Furman v. Georgia, the "guilt" phase of petitioner's trial is to be followed by a separate sentencing proceeding in which the jury is directed to answer three statutorily prescribed questions. One of these questions – and the only question of relevance here – directed the jury to determine whether there is "a probability that the defendant would commit criminal acts of violence that would constitute a continuing threat to society." The jury's affirmative response to this question resulted in Mr. Barefoot being sentenced to death.

The principle evidence presented to the jury on the question of petitioner's "future dangerousness" was the expert testimony of two psychiatrists, Dr. John T. Holbrook and Dr. James Grigson, both of whom testified for the prosecution.

Over defense counsel's objection, the prosecution psychiatrists were permitted to offer clinical opinions regarding Mr. Barefoot, including their opinions on the ultimate issue of future dangerousness, even though they had not performed a psychiatric examination or evaluation of him. Instead, the critical psychiatric testimony was elicited through an extended hypothetical question propounded by the prosecutor.

On the basis of the assumed facts stated in the hypothetical, both Dr. Holbrook and Dr. Grigson gave essentially the same testimony.

First, the petitioner (Mr. Barefoot) was diagnosed as a severe criminal sociopath, a label variously defined as describing persons who "lack a conscience," and who "do things which serve their own purposes without regard for any consequences or outcomes to other people." Second, both psychiatrists testified that petitioner would commit criminal acts of violence in the future. Dr. Holbrook stated that he could predict petitioner's future behavior in this regard "within reasonable psychiatric certainty." Dr. Grigson was more confident, claiming predictive accuracy of "one hundred percent and absolute."

James Grigson was featured prominently in Barefoot v. Estelle and the corresponding American Psychiatric Association Amicus brief. He played the same role repeatedly in the Texas legal system. For over three decades before his retirement in 2003, he would testify, when requested at death sentence hearings, to a high certainty as to "whether there is a probability that the defendant would commit criminal acts of violence that would constitute a continuing threat to society." An affirmative answer by the sentencing jury imposed the death penalty automatically, as it was on Thomas Barefoot, who was executed on October 30, 1984.

James Grigson was expelled in 1995 from the American Psychiatric Association and the Texas Association of Psychiatric Physicians for two chronic ethics violations: making statements in testimony on defendants he had not actually examined, and for predicting violence with 100% certainty. The press gave him the nickname of "Dr. Death."

The unreliability of psychiatric predictions of long-term future dangerousness is by now an established fact within the profession. In the early 1970s the American Psychiatric

Association appointed a Task Force of distinguished psychiatric experts "to assemble the body of knowledge concerning the individual violent patient and the clinical issues surrounding his case." The primary finding of this Task Force was that judgments concerning the long-run potential for future violence and the "dangerousness" of a given individual are "fundamentally of very low reliability." The report flatly concluded, "The state of the art regarding predictions of violence is very unsatisfactory. The ability of psychiatrists . . . (to) reliably predict future violence is unproved.

This conclusion has apparently been confirmed repeatedly by the research in the field, including research designed to establish the validity of psychiatric predictions of violent behavior. A 1975 monograph published by the National Institute of Mental Health, determined that the professional literature demonstrated no reliable criteria for psychiatric predictions of long-term future criminal behavior.

A more recent monograph, also published by the National Institute of Mental Health, again found that psychiatrists were more often wrong than right in predicting violent behavior over an extended period of time (Monahan, 1981). After a review of all major research published in the 1970s, the monograph concluded that no psychiatric procedures or techniques had succeeded in reducing the high rate of "false positive" predictions—that is, affirmative predictions of future violent behavior that are subsequently proven erroneous. Professor Monahan observed that, even allowing for possible distortions in certain of the research data, "it would be fair to conclude that the best clinical research currently in existence indicates that psychiatrists and psychologists are accurate in no more than one out of three predictions of violent behavior over a several-year period. . . ."

10.2 Correct no more than one out of three times!

How is this possible? We note that in the last seven years there were fewer than 10 million violent crimes committed in the United States. This represents less than a 3% chance of a randomly chosen person committing one. Thus simply predicting, "they won't" would be right 97% of the time. So why are psychiatrists so far wrong? Obviously they are not predicting for the general population.

A closer look begins to shed light on the subject. We can think of the data as part of a three-factor design. Factor 1 is the psychiatrist concluding that the defendant will or will not commit further mayhem. Factor 2 is the decision to release the defendant or not. And Factor 3 is the outcome, does the defendant commit further crimes or not? What we observe is only what happens when the defendant is released. When not released we do not know what would have happened had they had the opportunity to do ill. Within the observed data cells we find that when a defendant is predicted to be law-abiding the recidivism rate is but 1 time in 12. But in the cell where the defendant is predicted to continue to do bad things the recidivism rate is 1 in 3. Thus it is only for this one cell that the psychiatrist is wrong 2/3 of the time. To calculate overall accuracy we must look at all of the cells in the design and somehow figure out how to deal with the missing data.

But we must still wonder why are psychiatrists wrong a majority of the time even in just that one cell? One can easily see that simply by saying that the defendant will not recidivate the accuracy could immediately improve (at least in the observed data) to being right two-thirds of the time. Why would psychiatrists continue to behave in a way that makes them look bad, especially when improvement is so easy? Is it because psychiatrists are not statisticians? Or is there some other reason?

The answer, we believe, is that there is an asymmetric loss function. Just as weather forecasters in the Midwest tend to substantially over-predict the appearance of tornados, so too do psychiatrists seem to view the release of a potentially dangerous person as an error of greater consequence than the continued incarceration of a possibly safe one. This is surely not the only kind of loss function that could be chosen; Moses Maimonides, the famous 12th century sage, said that it would be preferable to free 1,000 guilty persons than to punish a single innocent one. At least some modern psychiatrists apparently have a loss function that tilts sharply away from the direction favored by Maimonides.[4]

Such problems are not unique to psychiatric prediction. A canonical medical example of this type manifests itself in the treatment of suspected appendicitis. In one moderately large study (Graff et al., 2000), 1,026 patients presented with signs and symptoms that might be interpreted as being caused by appendicitis. Of these, 110 patients (10.5%) turned out to be false positives and had their appendices removed unnecessarily. Of the 916 remaining patients, all of whom actually had appendicitis, 170 (18.6%) were false negatives. The total error rate was 29%. Note that there was half again as many false negatives as false positives, which reflects a cost function that suggests the physicians were exercising caution in putting patients through surgery unnecessarily. The risks of unnecessary surgery are well known. The risks of the false negatives involved increased chances of such complications as abscess formation and perforation[5]. Managing these competing risks can only be accomplished by using outcome data to determine the appropriate loss function. But as we have shown, we can assess what the *de facto* loss function is from the observed outcomes.

10.3 Conclusions

It is easy to decry a prediction that is taken out of context. Interpreting the statistic quoted that psychiatrists are wrong 2/3 of the time to mean that psychiatrists don't know what they're doing is likely a mistake. First, they are probably not wrong globally 2/3 of the time, if we include how often they are right (11 out of 12) when they predict no recidivism. Also we have no knowledge of how often they are right or wrong when the defendants are not released from custody. This surely adds substantially to the uncertainty of our estimates of their accuracy.

Second, without an understanding of the character of the loss function, we do not know whether the predictions made are wise. How much worse is it to keep a harmless defendant in custody than to loose a dangerous one on society? This situation is not unique to psychiatrists and murderers, it manifests itself throughout medicine: should a cancerous prostate be removed? Should a pregnancy be terminated if there is the possibility of the fetus being seriously damaged? Or, in the simple example given here, should a suspect appendix be removed? In all of these situations we must know both how accurate are the predictions as well as the consequences of both kinds of errors.

Nothing in life is more than 3 to 1.

Damon Runyon

On the role of replication in the advance of science: The survival of the fittist

11.1 Introduction

The principal epistemological tenet of the paradigm for modern science is replicability, and was laid out by Francis Bacon in the early 17th century. Replicability begins with the idea that science is not private and so claims that are made by one person must be available to be tested by others. The way that this idea has grown over time starts with the recognition that initial investigations are almost always done on a small scale and hence they exhibit the variability inherent in small studies. What this means is that there will be results reported that are epiphenomenal, for example false positives. But, when such things appear in the scientific literature other investigators will rush to replicate. If the attempts to replicate don't pan out the initial result is brushed aside as the statistical anomaly it was and science moves on. Scientific tradition sets an initial acceptance criterion for much research that tolerates a fair number of false positives (typically, one time out of twenty) because:

(i) it is not practical to do preliminary research on any topic that is on a large enough scale to diminish the likelihood of statistical artifacts to truly tiny levels, and

(ii) it is more difficult to rediscover a true result that was previously dismissed because it failed to reach some stringent level of acceptability, than it would be to reject a false positive after subsequent work fails to replicate it.

This approach has meant that the scientific literature is littered with an embarrassing number of remarkable results that were later shown to be anomalous[1].

11.2 ESP in North Carolina

A wonderful example of this effect originated in the 1930s at Duke University. J. B. Rhine, a botanist turned parapsychologist, did psychic research looking for people with extra-sensory perception. He found one with Adam Linzmayer, an economics undergraduate at Duke. In the spring of 1931, as a volunteer in one of Rhine's experiments, Linzmayer was seen to perform far better than chance would suggest. In subsequent experiments Linzmayer's performance retreated back to chance. Rather than dismiss the initial finding, Rhine concluded that Linzmayer's "extra-sensory perception has gone through a marked decline." But the experimentation continued until Rhine encountered Hubert Pearce, who had a remarkable run of successes before he too succumbed to the loss of his psychic gift. But this spotty record of intermittent success did not deter the energetic Rhine from continuing. The University of Chicago researcher, Harold Gulliksen, wrote a scathing review of Rhine's 1934 opus *Extra-Sensory Perception*, suggesting that although the statistical methods that Rhine used were seriously flawed, he would not discuss them for fear that he would distract attention from the monumental errors in his experimental design[2].

Rhine's reaction to, and interpretation of, normal random (stochastic) variation provides an object lesson in how humans, even scientists, allow what they want to be true overwhelm objective good sense. Nobel Laureate Daniel Kahneman spends the 500 pages of his recent book *Thinking, Fast and Slow*, laying out how and why humans behave this way.

11.3 Shrinking effects in science

Alas, the shrinking of the size of scientific results is not a phenomenon confined to scientific exotica like ESP. It manifests itself everywhere and often leads the general public to wonder how much of the scientific literature can be believed. Recently John Ioanndis, a prominent epidemiologist published a paper with the provocative title "Why most published research findings are false." Despite this title, Ioanndis provides a thoughtful explanation of why research results are often not as dramatic as first thought, and then elaborates the characteristics of studies that control the extent to which their results shrink upon replication. This topic proves to be one that troubles more than scientists. The author Jonah Lehrer wrote a wide ranging essay in the *New Yorker* (Lehrer, 2010) whose broader point of view was well expressed by his title, "The truth wears off: Is there something wrong with the scientific method?"

None of Ioanndis' explanations came as a surprise to those familiar with statistics, which is, after all, the Science of Uncertainty. Larger studies with bigger sample sizes yield more stable results; studies in which there are great financial consequences may more often yield biases; when study designs are flexible results vary more. There is also a bias due to publication policies of scientific journals. Let me illustrate with a generic, but still hypothetical, example.

Let us assume that we are doing a trial for some sort of medical treatment. Further, suppose that although the treatment has no effect (perhaps the medical equivalent of an ESP study) it seems on its face to be a really good idea. To make this more concrete, suppose modern scientific methods were available and trusted in the 19th century, and someone decided to use them to test the efficacy of using leeches[3] to draw blood and so balance the bodily humors and thence cure fevers. If but a single study was done the odds are it would find no effect. If, over a long period of time, many such studies were done, we might find that most would find no effect, a fair number might show a small negative effect, and an equal number a small positive effect, all this quite by chance. But chance, being what it is, if there are enough studies done, a few would show a substantial positive effect (and be balanced by a similar number that showed complementary negative effects). The big picture can be depicted as in Figure 11.1.

Of course, if we were privy to such a big picture summary, we could see immediately that the treatment has no efficacy and is merely showing random variation. But having such a comprehensive view has not been possible in the past (although there is currently a push to build a database that would produce such plots for all treatments being studied—the Cochrane Collaboration). Instead what happens

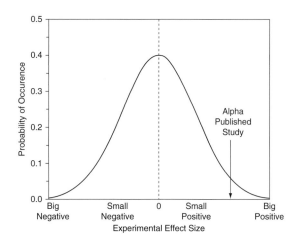

Figure 11.1

is that researchers who do a study and find no significant effect cannot publish it, for editors want to save the scarce room in their journals for research that finds something. Thus studies with null, or small, estimates of treatment effects are either thrown away, or placed in some sort of metaphorical file drawer.

But if someone gets lucky, and does a study whose results, quite by chance, falls further out in the tail of the normal curve, they let out a whoop of success, write it up, and get it published in some A-list journal; perhaps the *Journal of the American Medical Association*, or *The New England Journal of Medicine*. This is the alpha study. A publication in such a prestigious journal garners an increase in the visibility of both the research and the researcher—a win–win.

The attention generated by such a publication naturally leads to attempts to replicate; sometimes these replication studies turn out to have been done *before* the alpha study, lending support to the hypothesis that the alpha study might be anomalous. Typically these studies do not show an effect as large as was seen in the alpha study. Moreover the replication studies are not published in the A-list journals, for they are not path breaking. They appear in more minor outlets, if they are accepted for publication at all.

And so a pattern emerges. A startling and wonderful result appears in the most prestigious journals and news of the finding is trumpeted in the media. Subsequently, independent studies also appear, but few see them, and fewer still are picked up by the media to diminish the thoughts of a break-through generated by the alpha study. But sometimes news of diminished efficacy percolates out to the field and perhaps even the public at large. And then we start to worry, "does any treatment really work?"

One version of this effect has come to be called "the Tower of Babel" bias (Gregoire et al. 1995). Referring to significant findings published in international journals with wide readership. Studies whose research yields results that either do not achieve statistical significance, or show only a small effect, either publish in local journals, or not at all. Thus international estimates of treatment effects thus tend to have a positive bias.

11.4 Things are different in China

The stage is now set for us to shift our gaze to research done in the often-mysterious East. Chinese medical research is almost invisible to western scientists, but the reverse is not true. Chinese medical researchers are well aware of the major findings in the West, although they are likely less familiar with the more minor publications. So with the background of shrinking effect sizes over time firmly in hand, let us hypothesize what we might find if we were to look carefully at the findings of Chinese medical researchers as they strive to replicate Western medical findings on a Chinese population. The Chinese researchers are well aware of the results of the various alpha studies, so, when they try to replicate those studies we would expect to find the same shrinkage of effect sizes on replication that are the rule in the West. Is this what happens?

Zhenglun Pan and his team of international scholars did a large meta-analysis[4] of dozens of studies done in China that were meant to be replications of earlier studies. They then redid the same meta-analysis with studies from other Asian (but non-Chinese) researchers, as well as non-Asian, non-Chinese researchers. They found that Chinese studies in several different areas, although primarily focused on genetic epidemiology, seemed to find effect sizes at, or surpassing, those found in the alpha study. The authors termed this a 'reverse Tower of Babel' bias. Although this bias was the largest in Chinese studies, it was also found, to a lesser extent, in non-Chinese Asian research. Replications on the same subject by non-Chinese, non-Asian researchers found the smallest effect sizes of all.

Figures 11.2 and 11.3 show a graphic summary of Pan et al.'s meta-analyses. An odds ratio of one means that the effect of the treatment is the same as that of the control (placebo).

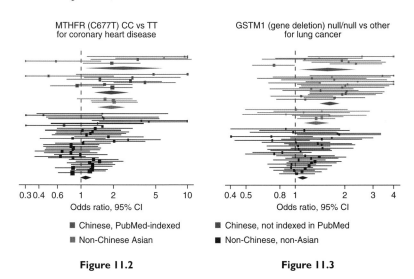

Figure 11.2   Figure 11.3

11.5 What have we learned?

Science is designed to be self-correcting. Attempts to replicate the science provide evidence that it has gone astray. Or at least that's the theory. The real world, filled with fallible people and institutions, practically guarantees that the path toward progress meanders, sometimes massively. But this is not all bad. As David Deutsch has emphasized, the evolution of a scientific idea is different from the Darwinian evolution of an organism in at least two important ways.

First, ideas evolve in ways that are directed by the intelligence of the investigators. Contrast this with biological evolution, which has no goal other than maximizing the likelihood of that particular mixture of genes spreading.

Second, if a particular phenotype[5] emerges that cannot survive, it becomes an evolutionary dead-end, but an idea that is a failure can still have parts that can be retrieved and subsequently used.

The story told here provides some compelling examples, if any were needed, that the road to improvement has potholes of misinformation and twists of political intrigue. But so long as we maintain a healthy skepticism, and remain free to publicly question the status quo, we shall continue to advance—at least for those disciplines for which the direction of an advance is known. To borrow Julian Jaynes' evocative metaphor, the physical and biological sciences are like a mountain in which the direction of advancement is clear. It is upward. Of course there are periods of confusion, but they are on the ledges, never in the overall direction. Things are different in the humanities and, perhaps, to some extent, even the social sciences, which are more like a forest, in full shining summer, with paths criss-crossing, some wide with fashion, others overgrown with disuse. It is direction that is wanting, not altitude. And the pitons and ropes so critical for ascending a mountain are replaced with blinders and earplugs as people wander the forest shouting "follow me, this is the way." This metaphor may help to explain why the scientific method, so powerful in hard sciences, fails when applied to subjects in which there is no clear idea of what constitutes an advance.

We live in the real world, where what we see should not be taken at face value—even 'objective science.' Every scientific study carries along with its results some sense of its own credibility. Studies with larger sample sizes are more credible than those that are smaller, ceteris paribus. If those doing the study have a great deal riding on the result credibility suffers. We must always be vigilant. But the current, flawed, system of independent studies being used to test results obtained by someone else, is the best available, although as flaws are detected in the system we can institute reforms. Such reforms always move in the direction of greater openness and greater accessibility to the raw data from which the conclusions are drawn.

The success of the scientific method thus relies on the continued existence and prosperity of researchers who relentlessly fit experimental data to theory. In a phrase, the validity of science depends on the survival of the fittists.

Another Hindrance to Progress

Introduction

The problem is never how to get new, innovative thoughts into your mind, but how to get old ones out.

Dee Hock[1]

At a 2010 conference dealing with the role of evidence in medicine, an emergency room physician complained about the frequent necessity of making a diagnosis without having as much evidence as he would minimally need to do so with some confidence. But he recognized that this is the nature of emergency room medicine—decisions (as distinct from conclusions) must be made quickly, for delays may place the patient at additional risk. So this was not his complaint. What he was upset about was that his diagnosis was then acted upon as if it were true, and was rarely modified even if the amount of subsequent evidence favoring another diagnosis far outweighed the amount of evidence used for the initial diagnosis.

A second researcher, who had gathered data examining this issue, confirmed this observation. But then he added to it by saying that the excessive inertia of the initial diagnosis remained both when the case was "handed off" to another physician, and when the original physician continued with it.

This vexing tendency for decisions to carry more inertia than the weight of their generating evidence is not confined to medicine. It pervades all aspects of our lives and has been carefully studied by psychologists. They call this the "Confirmation Bias," and define it as a tendency for people to prefer information that confirms their preconceptions or hypotheses, independently of whether they are true.[2] It describes when people reinforce their existing attitudes by selectively collecting new evidence, by interpreting evidence in a biased way or by selectively recalling information from memory that supports the point of view that they currently hold.[3]

The slow adoption of evidence-based science may only be partially due to the difficulty of discarding well-beloved practices simply because data do not support them. There is another impediment—the power of convention. The research surrounding such concepts as confirmation bias helps to explain the inertia that is a psychological and social force as much as a physical one. The Newtonian axiom that bodies in place tend to stay in place unless acted upon by an outside force has a psychological parallel. Einstein's remark that "old ideas never die, just the people who believe them," emphasizes this point.[4] Thus it seems fitting to conclude this book with a brief examination of some developments that promised to be substantial improvements over conventional practice.

In Chapter 12 I will describe two developments that have not yet fully caught on. One, the use of checklists in medicine is new and promises a real reduction in medical errors. The second, hand-washing, is a practice whose efficacy in preventing infection was convincingly demonstrated more than 150 years old, yet is still not fully operational. Chapter 13 takes a broader view of the power of convention, examining three very different areas of application, where the superiority of an unconventional approach is established and yet the status quo remained. Chapter 13 is an appropriate place to end, for it leaves us with hope. Two of the innovations discussed have not yet been adopted, but the third has been. The fact that it took almost four-hundred years for adoption splashes the cold water of reality on enthusiastic reformers.

It is daunting to learn how difficult it has been for innovations to be adopted and illustrates once again Einstein's wisdom and the importance of patience. More than 150 years ago a sense of cautious optimism was emphasized by John Stuart Mill, implying that the long-run outlook is positive, but not necessarily rapid.

It is a piece of idle sentimentality that truth, merely as truth, has any inherent power denied to error of prevailing against the dungeon and the stake. Men are not more zealous for truth than they often are for error, and a sufficient application of legal or even social penalties will generally succeed in stopping the propagation of either.

The real advantage which truth has consists in this, that when an opinion is true, it may be extinguished once, twice or many times, but in the course of ages there will generally be found persons to rediscover it, until some one of its reappearances fall on a time when from favorable circumstances it escapes persecution until it has made such headway as to withstand all subsequent attempts to suppress it.

John Stuart Mill, *On Liberty* (1859, Chapter 2)

CHAPTER 12

What does it take to change practice?

Many are stubborn in pursuit of the path they have chosen, few in pursuit of the goal.

Fredrick Nietzsche

12.1 Introduction[1]

On Saturday June 5, 2010 in Yankee stadium, 20,272 fans watched Miguel Cotto defeat the WBA super welterweight champion Yuri Foreman. It was Foreman's first loss. Two days before the fight began the Yankees had a home game against the Baltimore Orioles, which ran late. Standing anxiously at the sidelines during the game was Brad Jacobs. It was Jacobs' responsibility to transform the stadium from a venue built for baseball to one suitable for a championship boxing match. To accomplish this he had the aid of 200 workers who had to erect a 60-foot-high canopy over a ring as well as install 6,000 folding chairs on the field of Yankee Stadium. It was a large and complex task with a tight deadline and no room for error. When queried about how he would accomplish this impressive transformation Jacobs tapped on a three-inch-thick loose-leaf binder that he pulled from his briefcase. It was a catalog of every last detail needed to transform Yankee Stadium into a boxing arena for the first time. It included a monstrous check-list.

The practice of using a check-list to aid in reducing errors in a complex task did not originate with Brad Jacobs. In his now famous *New Yorker* article

"The Check-list" Atul Gawande (Gawande, 2007) relates the story of Boeing's Model 299—on the eve of World War II it was the leading candidate to be the US military's next long-range bomber. On October 30, 1935 a cadre of Army brass was gathered at Wright Air Field in Dayton, Ohio to see the Model 299 being put through its paces. In Gawande's words,

the plane roared down the tarmac, lifted off smoothly, and climbed sharply to three hundred feet. Then it stalled, turned on one wing, and crashed in a fiery explosion.

The subsequent investigation concluded that the crash was due to "pilot error." But the pilot, Major Ployer P. Hill (who died in the crash) was the US Army Air Corps' chief of flight testing, and was very experienced. What went wrong? The 299 was considerably more complex than previous aircraft.

The new plane required the pilot to attend to the four engines, a retractable landing gear, new wing flaps, electric trim tabs that needed adjustment to maintain control at different airspeeds, and constant-speed propellers whose pitch had to be regulated with hydraulic controls, among other features. While doing all this, Hill had forgotten to release a new locking mechanism on the elevator and rudder controls.

Perhaps, as one newspaper put it, it was "too much airplane for one man to fly."

Not willing to give up on what was an otherwise extraordinary aircraft, a group of test pilots got together and considered what to do.

They came up with an ingeniously simple approach: they created a pilot's checklist, with step-by-step checks for takeoff, flight, landing, and taxiing. Its mere existence indicated how far aeronautics had advanced. In the early years of flight, getting an aircraft into the air might have been nerve-racking, but it was hardly complex. Using a checklist for takeoff would no more have occurred to a pilot than to a driver backing a car out of the garage. But this new plane was too complicated to be left to the memory of any pilot, however expert.

With the checklist in hand, the pilots went on to fly the Model 299 a total of 1.8 million miles without one accident. The Army ultimately ordered almost thirteen thousand of the aircraft, which it dubbed the B-17.

12.2 Checklists and medical care

"Medicine today has entered its B-17 phase. Substantial parts of what hospitals do— most notably, intensive care—are now too complex for clinicians to carry them out reliably from memory alone. Intensive-care life support has become too much medicine for one person to fly."

Intensive-care medicine has become the art of managing extreme complexity. The average stay of an intensive-care patient is four days, and the survival rate is eighty-six per cent. In 1997 Israeli scientists published a study of patients in intensive-care units who were observed for twenty-four-hour periods.

They found that the average patient required a hundred and seventy-eight individual actions per day, ranging from administering a drug to suctioning the lungs, and every one of them posed risks. Remarkably, the nurses and doctors were observed to make an error in just one per cent of these actions—but that still amounted to an average of two errors a day with every patient. Intensive care succeeds only when we hold the odds of doing harm low enough for the odds of doing good to prevail.

Treating a human is different than flying an airplane. All planes of a specific type are more-or-less identical. A checklist can be prepared and we can expect that it will be appropriate for any particular plane of that type. And, while all humans share the same core structures, the interaction of a particular type of illness or injury with a specific person, can yield unique features. Is there enough commonality to make a checklist possible, let alone useful?

Peter Pronovost, a critical-care specialist at Johns Hopkins thought so. He had seen how all too often infections arose when intravenous lines were inserted, and believed that such complications could be reduced with a little more care. So in 2001 he developed a simple checklist of five steps doctors ought to take to avoid infections when inserting a line:

1 Wash their hands with soap.
2 Clean the patient's skin with chlorhexidine antiseptic.
3 Put sterile drapes over the entire patient.
4 Wear a sterile mask, hat, gown and gloves.
5 Put a sterile dressing over the catheter site once the line is in.

There was nothing revolutionary about this list. It has long been taught in medical school as standard procedure. Nevertheless, Pronovost wrote down this list and asked surgical nurses at Johns Hopkins to record how often doctors completed each step when they inserted a line. In one month he found that in one third of the patients at least one step had been skipped.

The following month nurses were authorized by the hospital administration to stop doctors if they saw them skipping a step on the checklist and have them remediate it immediately. The results were so remarkable that no statistical analysis was needed to measure the checklist's efficacy. In the year following, the ten-day line-infection rate dropped from eleven percent to zero. In a fifteen month follow-on study only two line infections occurred over the entire period.

Compared with prior experience at this one hospital, adherence to this simple checklist had prevented forty-three infections and eight deaths. It also saved two million dollars in costs.

After this original success Pronovost traveled widely, describing the results he obtained at Johns Hopkins to an average of seven cities a month. He found little enthusiasm for checklists. Tom Piskorowski, an intensive care physician at Sinai-Grace Hospital in Detroit echoed the opinions of many when he said, "Forget the paperwork. Take care of the patient."

Nevertheless, Blue Cross Blue Shield of Michigan was persuaded to give hospitals a small bonus for participating in Pronovost's checklist program. This became known as the Keystone Initiative, the results of which were published in the *New England Journal of Medicine* in December of 2006. Within the first three months the infection rate in participating hospitals fell 66%. Typical intensive care units, including the ones at Sinai-Grace, cut their quarterly infection rates to zero. In the first 18 months they estimated that the participating hospitals saved $175 million and more than 1,500 lives. The successes of checklists have continued since.

Yet the use of checklists in medicine has not become universal; not even close. In a recent interview Pronovost was asked how long before the average doctor or nurse is as apt to have a checklist in their hand as a stethoscope. He replied, "At the current rate, it will never happen. The fundamental problem with the quality of American medicine is that we've failed to view delivery of health care as a science."

The National Institutes of Health has over a $30 billion/year budget. Pronovost estimates that it would take only two to three million dollars to do for all of the United States what has already been done for Michigan. "It could be done within two years if the country wanted it."

Peter Pronovost's frustration and impatience is palpable. He has demonstrated convincingly how something as simple and inexpensive as checklists can yield dramatic improvements in medical care and impressive savings in both human lives and treasure. Yet despite this evidence more than a decade has passed and we are a long way from universal acceptance.

I fear that optimism will not be helped when we examine the speed of adoption of earlier innovations.

12.3 Hand washing in 19th century Vienna

On July 1, 1846 the Hungarian physician Ignac Semmelweis was appointed head resident at the First Obstetrical Clinic of the Vienna General Hospital (Nuland, 2003). There were two clinics at the hospital: Clinic 1, staffed by doctors, and Clinic 2, staffed by midwives. Both clinics provided obstetrical services to indigent women. In return for free services the women agreed to serve as training vehicles for the doctors and midwives. The maternal mortality rate, due to what was then called Puerperal Fever[2], was horrific but far worse at Clinic 1 than at Clinic 2 (see Figure 12.1). Obviously there were wild fluctuations over time, but because women were assigned to one clinic or the other more-or-less at random[3] it was truly a puzzle why, despite the parallel fluctuations, the results were always so much worse at Clinic 1.

The women of Vienna knew about the differences between the two clinics and would work hard to get themselves admitted to the safer Clinic 2. They were so fearful of Clinic 1 that some women preferred to give birth on the street. They would then tell the admissions office that they had given birth en route to the hospital, so that they would still be eligible for free child care benefits. The puzzle about Clinic 1 grew more profound when it was discovered that the incidence of Puerperal Fever among street births was closely akin to that in Clinic 2.

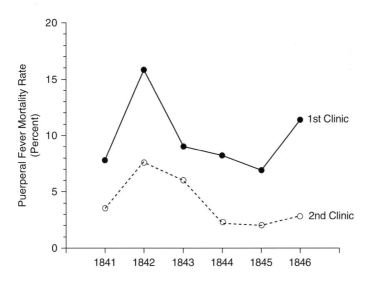

Figure 12.1 Pueperal fever annual mortality rates at the Vienna General Hospital.

The consistent poor showing of Clinic 1 troubled Semmelweis profoundly and his uncovering that it was safer to give birth on the street than in Clinic 1, with a physician's assistance, only added emphasis. The pathway to the resolution of the problem was illuminated by a tragedy.

In 1847 Semmelweis' friend and colleague, Jakob Kolletschka was nicked by a student's scalpel while performing a postmortem examination. Kolletschka subsequently died of an infection whose pathology showed remarkable similarity to those of women who died from Puerperal Fever. Semmelweis immediately saw a connection between the transmission of Puerperal Fever and cadaveric contamination. He concluded that it was "cadaverous particles" carried from the autopsy room to the delivery room that was the cause of the high incidence of Puerperal Fever in Clinic 1. This explanation neatly explained why the midwives in Clinic 2, who had no contact with corpses, had much better results.

Although there had been various theories of germs fulminating at the borders of science for centuries[4] there was little in the way of formal proof and general acceptance until Pasteur's famous paper "The Germ Theory and its applications to medicine and surgery," which he read before the French Academy of Sciences

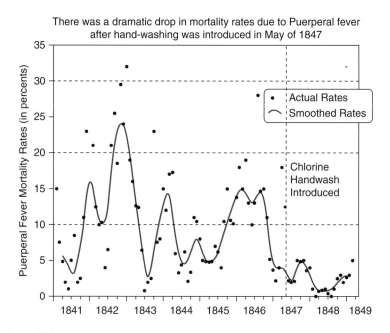

Figure 12.2 Pueperal mortality rates at the Vienna General Hospital from 1841 through 1849.

in the April of 1878. But despite this Semmelweis felt that whatever it was that was being carried into the birthing area, improvements in outcome would likely be made if physicians washed their hands before delivering a baby. He instituted a policy requiring that this be done using a solution of chlorinated lime. He settled on this because this same solution had been successful in removing the putrid smell of infected autopsy tissue.

Semmelweis' hand washing policy went into effect in May 1847 and the mortality rates due to Puerperal Fever dropped immediately from 18% in April to 2% in June. The monthly mortality rates before and after the intervention are shown dramatically in Figure 12.2.

12.2 Hand washing in 20th century America

We have seen that while there is a great deal of evidence emerging of the efficacy of checklists to reduce errors in medical practice, the use of checklists is a very long way from universal. Indeed despite the strenuous efforts of Peter Pronovost to spread the gospel of checklists their adoption has been disappointingly slow. Atul Gawande has opined that "If a new drug was as effective at savings lives as Peter Pronovost's checklists, there would be a nationwide campaign urging doctors to use it." To assess the speed of adoption it seems helpful to compare it to something[5]. Hand washing seems an apt choice.

To my eye, it has been more than a century and a half since Ignac Semmelweis showed pretty conclusively that by having physicians simply wash their hands between patients there would be wonderful improvements in patient outcome. Yes, it was just for one specific kind of infection, but it doesn't take much of an intuitive jump to infer that it would work for many other kinds as well. Moreover, what is the downside? Who is harmed if physicians wash more often than they need to? A policy of washing hands between patients seems a complete no-brainer. So let us jump forward 150 years and see how close to universal adoption this simple policy has achieved.

In the Spring of 2001, *Emerging Infectious Diseases*, a publication of the Centers for Disease Control, published an article by the Swiss physician Didier Pittet, which summarized the findings of about a dozen previous studies on the frequency of ICU physicians washing their hands before examining a patient. These studies were published between 1981 and 1999. An extract from that summary is in Table 12.1.

TABLE 12.1 **Compliance with hand hygiene in intensive care units**

Year	Average Compliance
1981	30%
1981	41%
	28%
1983	32%
1987	81%
1990	51%
1990	29%
1991	40%
1992	40%
1999	36%
Median	*38%*

These results do not suggest optimism.

Pittet observed,

Noncompliance was higher in ICUs than in internal medicine, during procedures with a high risk for bacterial contamination, and when intensity of patient care was high."

In other words, compliance with hand washing worsened when the demand for hand cleansing was high . . . the lowest compliance rate (36%) was found in ICUs, where indications for hand washing were typically more frequent. The highest compliance rate (59%) was observed in pediatrics.

He also reported that when hand-washing directives were complied with there was a significant reduction in hospital infections and methicilllin-resistant *Staphylococcus aureus* (MRSA) cross-transmission rates over a 4-year period.

A revealing, albeit somewhat anecdotal, result comes from Brobson Lutz, an Infectious Disease Specialist in New Orleans. Dr. Lutz took several residents with him to a convention on infectious diseases. He stationed them in the restrooms adjacent to the meeting rooms and had them observe and record the frequency with which attendees at the convention washed their hands upon leaving the restroom. He found that, "Overall, only 68% of those observed washed their hands. Female meeting attendees (87%) were more likely to wash their hands in a public restroom than their male counterparts (56%)."

12.4 What can be done?

So far the prospects for improving the practice of medicine seem limited. Although no one questions the connection between hand washing and patient safety, there is considerable variation in opinion on how to increase compliance. In a very long and very complete 2009 report on improving compliance there were many studies cited and many suggestions made, but a key component in most of the strategies was (drum roll—wait for it—here it comes) the use of checklists! Alas, it is turtles all the way down[6].

Perhaps we need to think more creatively. One suggested path is provided by the search for an effective treatment of peptic ulcers. It was long thought that such ulcers were caused by stress, alcohol and spicy food. Most treatment was palliative and patients were asked to modify their lifestyle to cut back on drinking and reduce both stress and spicy food. Another alternative was provided by John Lykoudis, a Greek physician who, as early as 1958, was successful in treating patients for peptic ulcers with antibiotics. This was long before it was commonly recognized that bacteria were a dominant cause for the disease. This treatment went nowhere.

The causal role that the bacteria *Helicobacter pylori* played in peptic ulcers was rediscovered in 1982 by two Australian scientists, Robin Warren and Barry Marshall. In their original paper, Warren and Marshall contended that most stomach ulcers and gastritis were caused by colonization with this bacterium, not by stress, alcohol or spicy food.

This result was poorly received. In an attempt to provide a dramatic demonstration of the validity of their hypothesis Marshall drank a Petri dish containing a culture of organisms extracted from a patient suffering from a peptic ulcer. He soon developed gastritis. All of the bacteria, and the associated symptoms, disappeared after he took antibiotics. This self-experiment was published in 1985 in the *Australian Medical Journal* and has become among that journal's most cited articles.

In 1997 various governmental agencies, academic institutions, and the pharmaceutical industry launched a national education campaign to inform health care providers and consumers about the link between *H. pylori* and ulcers. This campaign reinforced the news that ulcers are a curable infection, and that antibiotics are an effective treatment.

In 2005, Marshall and Warren were awarded the Nobel Prize in Medicine "for their discovery of the bacterium *Helicobacter pylori* and its role in gastritis and peptic ulcer disease."

It is hard to know what role Marshall's self-experiment played in getting their discovery implemented. I suspect that the proximal cause of the widespread implementation of the new treatment was the broad campaign waged to inform both the professional and lay public. Perhaps his dramatic experiment played an important role in getting that campaign started. But it also suggests that in the modern world of lightning fast and wide-spread electronic communication we might be able to see effective reform if:

(i) there were a website listing hospitals that have implemented the rigorous use of checklists,

(ii) the equivalent of "secret shoppers" were used to estimate the frequency of hand washing among physicians[7], and those results were on a widely publicized web-site, and

(iii) health insurers took a page from Michigan Blue Cross Blue Shield and offered cash rewards for medical institutions that follow specified "best-practices" (or refused coverage at institutions that don't).

It would be a mistake to claim that medicine stands alone in its remarkable resistance to change. In the next chapter we broaden our view and so recognize that such inertia is an integral part of the human psyche.

CHAPTER 13

Why is a raven like a writing desk? Musing on the power of convention

As I compose this chapter[1], the writing desk I am using is a spanking new Macintosh laptop with many gigabytes of storage and enormous computing power. Its screen is a marvel of full-color clarity; it has a built-in video camera and microphone, and hence allows multiple methods of input and output. Yet it has a QWERTY keyboard. Why QWERTY?

The QWERTY keyboard, named for the order of the keys on the left side of the first row of letter keys, was invented in 1864 by Christopher Sholes, a Milwaukee newspaper editor. Its purpose was to split up keys that were commonly hit serially so that a too fast typist would not jam the associated type bars. In addition to its primary goal of slowing things down, it also aided left-handed English language typists, for far more words can be typed with only the keys under the left hand than under the right.

Now, since its purpose has long been anachronistic, why do we still persist in using it? The reason is, of course, the power of convention. After it became the conventional keyboard layout, and touch typists learned it they were loath to give it up and learn a different system, even if the newer system was demonstrably superior. And so now, almost 150 years later, QWERTY has survived; and, because virtually all subsequent generations learn to type using it, the likelihood of its being improved remains small.

In his 1801 *Statistical Breviary,* William Playfair, the Scot who invented many forms of statistical graphics proposed the pie chart. Playfair's pie had but three segments and showed what proportions of the Turkish Empire were in Europe, Asia and Africa. It worked very well. Indeed, to test its efficacy, one can easily demonstrate that a small child can tell that 1/3 is larger than 1/4 from a pie chart far more easily than from the fractions themselves. But since Playfair's time, pie charts have become conventional and thus often used to display information that is much more complex than is suitable for it, this despite strong evidence that pie chart's efficacy in such a situation is suspect.

In 1990, the New York Times used a pie very much like the one shown in Figure 13.1 to communicate the content of what New Yorkers typically discard. The content is a remarkably apt metaphor for the quality of the plot.

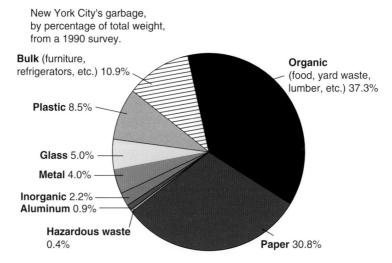

Figure 13.1 Pie chart of New York City's garbage.

We can tell how much of each component is discarded, but only by reading the amount from the label. Because we must "read" the graph rather than "see" it, it is natural to ask what is the value-added of the pictorial representation over the numerical. Such concerns as these led the statistician William Cleveland, in his 1985 book *The Elements of Graphing Data,* to propose the dot chart as an alternative. He found, through a series of experiments, that humans could visually judge lengths far more accurately than areas or angles, and so by transforming the pie segments to line segments punctuated with a large dot (see Figure 13.2), he was able to produce a plot that has substantially better perceptual characteristics than Playfair's pie. Nevertheless, in the intervening 25 years the popularity of the overmatched pie has not decreased and, sadly, the use of Cleveland's excellent proposal has seen no substantial increase[2].

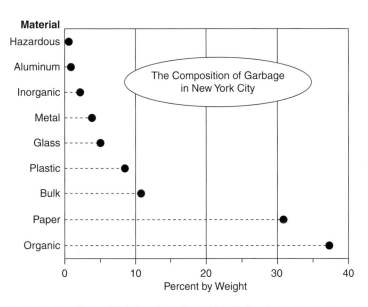

Figure 13.2 Dot chart of New York City's garbage.

Once again, the reason is convention.

It is natural to ask how long it takes for a genuinely superior product to supplant one that is well established? For the pie chart 20 years has not been enough; for the QWERTY keyboard it has been 150 years and we are still counting.

One would think that the speed with which convention is overturned depends strongly on how much of an improvement the unconventional technique provides, as well as how much evidence is available that supports the replacement. But the more carefully we look, the more evidence emerges that the path to improvement is littered with impediments that may take centuries to circumvent.

A powerful final example illustrates this and also provides the connection with the raven in the title.

까마귀, pronounced Ka-ma-gui, is the Korean word for raven, written in the remarkable Hangul alphabet. To understand the relevance of this example, we must go back almost six centuries. China's culture dominated Asia for centuries, and so it isn't surprising that the written Korean language of the 15th century used Chinese characters. Yet because the Korean language uses inflections and suffixes to add or modify meaning, whereas Chinese sentences are qualified in a different way, the use of Chinese characters was far from an ideal match. In addition, Chinese characters, known as *hanja*, were complex, numerous and so difficult to write that literacy was reserved for the aristocrats.

Sejong the Great, the fourth king of the Joseon Dynasty (1393–1910), apparently deplored the fact that common people, ignorant of the Chinese characters, were practically forced into illiteracy. He felt that this had important practical consequences, for they had no way of submitting grievances to the authorities for possible redress. Nor could they record their thoughts or experiences for posterity, placing obvious severe limits on the breadth of Korean science and art.

To ameliorate this situation, King Sejong set about creating an alphabet especially suited for the Korean language, and his success provided a remarkable model for others. It is far beyond the goals of this chapter to explain the details of the Hangul alphabet. Instead let me choose a few of its remarkable features.

First, it is completely phonetic. Thus, if you can already speak and understand the Korean language, all you need to do to be able to read and write is to memorize the symbols representing the 10 basic vowel sounds and the 14 basic consonant sounds. Apart from a few minor exceptions, the phonetic value of each symbol is invariant. Thus, any letter string, even if unfamiliar or nonsensical, can be sounded out instantly and accurately. There is no need to ever consult a dictionary for sounds or spellings. Contrast this with how the sound "f" is represented in English—fat, photo, laugh; how the same vowel, say "a," can have many different sounds—fat, farm, face, fall, hurrah; and some letters in English have no sound at all—*p*sa*l*m, indi*c*t.

Each Korean character usually consists of two or three components: ① a consonant + ② a vowel, ① or a consonant + ② a vowel + ③ a consonant. Thus, each Hangul character is of one syllable structured as:

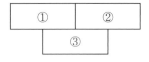

The table below (Diamond Sutra Recitation Group, 2004) lists the Hangul letters and their approximate pronunciation in English.

Consonants (① And ③)	Vowels (②)
ㄱ—G	ㅏ—A
ㄴ—N	ㅑ—YA
ㄷ—D	ㅓ—EUR
ㄹ—L	ㅕ—YUE
ㅁ—M	ㅜ—U
ㅂ—B	ㅠ—YU
ㅅ—S	ㅗ—O
ㅇ—A	ㅛ—YO
ㅈ—Z	ㅡ—UE
ㅊ—CH	ㅣ—I
ㅋ—K	
ㅌ—T	
ㅍ—P	
ㅎ—H	

To see how easy it is to spell and read in Hangul, consider the two-syllable word "Hangul" which is written 한글. Use the table above to sound out the written word.

Second, great effort was expended to aid memory. Each consonant sound is constructed to look like your mouth when you say it! In English, only one letter has this characteristic ("o"). In Hangul all consonants have this characteristic. Sometimes the letter looks like the shape of the mouth viewed from the front (e.g. ㅁ, the letter "mium," which is an "m" sound pronounced with the lips spaced a little apart). Often the letter is a stylized drawing of the mouth when looked at from the side after a vertical cut down the center of the head, where the location of the lips and tongue indicate the letter. For example, ㄴ, the letter "nium," an "n" sound, depicts the outline of the tongue touching the upper palate.

And the letter ㅅ "shiot," which, when pronounced, requires that the tip of the tongue and the upper teeth are brought close together, and sound is created by blowing through the narrowed passage.

In addition, the very names of the letters provide information on their pronunciation. So, for example, the letter "rial" ㄹ is pronounced as an "r" at the beginning of a syllable and as an "l" when it appears at the end of a syllable. Compare with mium, which has an "m" sound at both ends of a word.

It was generally agreed that a clever person could learn the entire alphabet in a morning and so go from illiterate to literate by lunchtime. Contrast this task with the 20th century Chinese requirement that children must learn at least 2,000 *hanja* characters by the end of high school to be considered appropriately literate.

It would seem that this remarkable innovation would be adopted rapidly, but alas the power of convention prevailed. Confucian scholars of the 15th century believed that *hanja* was the only legitimate writing system. Choi Manli, a senior scholar of the time, presented a petition to the king criticizing the new alphabet:

Since the new alphabet is so easily understood, I fear that the people will fall into laziness and never make efforts to learn. Those who do not use Chinese characters but other letters and alphabets, such as Mongols, Sohans, Jurchens, Japanese and Tibetans, are all barbarians without exception. To use new letters would make us barbarians ourselves.

He continued,

Why does Your Highness seek to alter a language that has been used since early antiquity and has no ill effects, and place alongside it a set of coarse and vulgar characters of no worth at all? Is not this script, moreover, a mere transcription of the words spoken by the peasants, without the slightest resemblance to the original Chinese Characters?

Despite opposition of this sort, Hangul's use as an official Korean alphabet grew in fits and starts, and it took fully 500 years before it became widely accepted as the Korean alphabet.

I hope that I have demonstrated that it is not unreasonable to believe that the inertia of convention acts as a drag on innovation. Yet simply recognizing this obstacle will not make the power of convention disappear, nor should it. When faced with a single communication task (e.g. reporting the results of an experiment in a research paper), we should first consider the conventional way to do it. If such an approach allows it to be done adequately, then that is a sensible path to follow; fighting convention can age you quickly. If, on the other hand, the task is but the first of many (e.g. writing the first of many national statistics reports, with many similar data sets—see Pickle et al. (1996)), the cost of fighting convention may be amortized over the long run.

What have we learned from these examples? It seems to me that QWERTY has little to recommend it, and various alternatives have already been proposed. August Dvorak, a professor of education at the University of Washington, patented one in 1936. The *Guiness Book of Records* tells us that Barbara Blackburn, the fastest typist on record (150 words/minute for 50 minutes, with peaks of 212 words/minute), set her record on a Dvorak keyboard. Obviously improvements are possible and some experiments in design should allow us to build on Dvorak's design. Implementing such an innovation is easy, since programmable keyboards can allow those whose touch-typing skills require QWERTY to keep it, but as we start teaching the new keyboard in schools, graduates who can perform better will transform the old keyboard to the new. One generation should just about do it.[3]

Pie charts have little to recommend them over Cleveland's dot charts; and, as soon as those who write graphic software replace pies with dots as the default option, we will see the end of this over-used invention.

The 15th century complaints from scholars about the ease of learning Hangul are surely relevant today. Yet one should not dissuade the Chinese and Japanese governments from considering the costs of keeping their ancient writing systems. Perhaps a Hangul-like Chinese keyboard might have more than 34 keys (24 letters + 10 numbers), but it would surely be far less cumbersome than current methods. If such an alphabet were invented and implemented, the two systems would probably operate in parallel for a while, for old ideas never really die, just the people who believe in them. But eventually offspring of King Sejong's marvelous Hangul alphabet would take over. Other languages have alternative phonetic alphabets (e.g. the Unifon alphabet is a way of writing English based on the principle of one letter per phoneme; it was created by John Malone in the 1930s) for other languages, but they have yet to overcome the power of convention. Still, the cost of maintaining the convention seems much smaller for English than Chinese.

And so, why is a raven like a writing desk? My answer is because both of them can be improved substantially, but the major part of the task is overcoming the inertia of convention and not inventing a superior product.

Afterword

This is an odd book—in some ways it is reminiscent of Stephen Leacock's young man who ran out of his house, jumped on his horse, and galloped off in all directions at once.

Its theme, if it has just one, is of illumination in both of its meanings. It is first about illumination in the sense of methods, ways of thinking, that provide light to allow us to understand better some aspects of the modern world of medicine. It follows the traditional view of illumination, of divine light, if we agree that studying the universe in an attempt to understand it is, in Maimonides' interpretation, akin to prayer. Thinking of epistemology in religious terms is not new. Galileo made the connection explicit in his oft quoted inference that "Mathematics is the language that God used to write the universe." Einstein followed the same metaphor with his conclusion that "God is subtle but not malicious."

It is also about illumination in a second sense, in which the understanding of our words and thoughts is clarified and enhanced through the inclusion of pictures. Modern illuminations differ in important ways from those that decorated medieval texts, but in their goals they are no more distant than second cousins.

The first section combines the two meanings explicitly, demonstrating how carefully chosen illuminations (statistical graphics) can communicate what we have found to others, but most importantly, to ourselves. It is this second aspect of data graphics that is the most exciting—forcing us to see what we had not expected. Exploratory analysis, using graphic displays, has become a critically important tool for every modern, empirical scientist. The second focus of this section is on illuminations as communicative devices connecting the often complex and arcane peaks on which resides much of modern science, to the regions, nearer sea level, where the mass of humanity live. Such displays need to be constructed carefully and clearly, keeping in mind the character of both the message and the recipients. I hope that the concerns that I expressed in the first chapter, of the dangers of communicating data that have been insufficiently processed, regardless of good intentions, are taken to heart. The other bits of advice on effective display in the other chapters are more specific, but I hope will be of value.

The second section of the book is meant to be illuminating in a different way. Yes, it too contains graphic displays of the empirical evidence, when I decided that they could be helpful, but the star of this part of the show is the combination of statistical thinking with a reverence for empiricism as a principal way of knowing things. The choice of topics within this section was purposely chosen to be eclectic, ranging among diagnosing hip fractures to judging the future behavior of felons to musing about the unexpectedly optimistic results of Chinese medical research. I chose this odd mixture to emphasize the generality of use for the methods being proposed. An important lesson that should be taken from this is that statistical thinking is both subtle and critically important. This is emphasized in Chapter 8, when we found that the efficacy of medical diagnostic procedures like the mammogram is far worse than our intuition would suggest. The difference between the probability that a mammogram is positive if one has cancer and the probability that a positive mammogram means that you have cancer, shocks one's intuition. It adds ammunition to John McCarthy's[1] well-known epigram "Do the math or forever be doomed to talk nonsense."

Finally, we concluded with two stories about the power of convention. People and institutions do not change quickly. But some inertia may be a good thing.[2] However, when solutions are needed urgently too much inertia may be harmful. In Chapter 12 I discuss some changes in medical procedures (checklists and hand washing) for which there is no viable alternative choice. And finally, in Chapter 13, I describe three very different kinds of inventions, whose superiority cannot be gainsaid, and yet resistance to their adoption continues.

The central idea that motivated everything in this book was stated clearly by the iconic physicist Richard P. Feynman:

For a successful technology, reality must take precedence over public relations, for nature cannot be fooled.

Feynman made this observation as part of his contribution to the report on the causes of the crash of the space shuttle *Challenger*. The decision to launch, despite the cold temperature, which was known to compromise the effectiveness of the O-rings crucial for success, was made because of political reasons to avoid further delay. Yet Feynman's wisdom is a long way from universally accepted.

In June of 2012, North Carolina business interests were concerned about the effect on the value of their beachfront properties and businesses if the prediction of a one-meter rise in the ocean are widely believed. To counter this, North Carolina's state legislature is considering a bill that would require the government to ignore new reports of the acceleration of rising sea levels and predictions of ocean and climate scientists. Business interests along the state's coastline encouraged lawmakers to include language in a law that would require future sea level estimates to be based only on data from past years. New evidence, especially on sea level rise that could be tied to global warming, would not be factored into the state's development plans for the coast.[3]

Not to be outdone by their neighbors, on May 31, 2012 the Alabama state legislature narrowly passed a law redefining π. The bill to change the value of π to exactly 3 was introduced without fanfare by Leonard Lee Lawson (R, Crossville), and rapidly gained support after a letter-writing campaign by members of the Solomon Society, a traditional values group. Governor Guy Hunt says he will sign it into law on Wednesday, June 6.

"I think mathematicians are being irrational, and it is time for them to admit it," said Lawson. "The Bible very clearly says in I Kings 7:23 that the altar font of Solomon's Temple was ten cubits across and thirty cubits in circumference, and that it was round in compass."

Lawson called into question the usefulness of any number that cannot be calculated exactly, and suggested that never knowing the exact answer could harm students' self-esteem. "We need to return to some absolutes in our society," he said, "the Bible does not say that the font was thirty-something cubits. Plain reading says thirty cubits. Period."[4]

It has been my hope that by explicating a number of situations in which we make decisions on the basis of evidence, instead of authority, we can make steady improvements. We must recognize that empirical evidence is sometimes complex and subtle and so I chose to emphasize the role that well-built graphical displays can play in aiding our understanding.

And this collaboration between evidence and graphic display can provide powerful illumination of any area. Today's topic was medicine; there are many others.

NOTES

PREFACE

1. Thanks to Edward Albee, who taught me this lesson explicitly in his famous one-act play *Zoo Story*.

INTRODUCTION

1. We might describe the old system as a physician's parallel to Ring Lardner's "'Shut up!' his father explained." But perhaps it could be more gently put as "Because I said so." How long gone are such notions.

2. My gratitude to my colleague Peter Scoles, who provided me with this wonderful example.

3. Louis, P. C. A. (1835). Recherches sur les effets de la saignée dans quelques maladies inflammatoires, et sur l'action de l'émétique et des vésicatoires dans la pneumonie. Paris: J-B Ballière.

4. In 1833 alone, France imported 42 million leeches for medical use (Ackerknecht, 1967, p. 62).

CHAPTER 1

1. *Brownfields,* for those unfamiliar with the term, are abandoned or underused properties, including industrial and commercial facilities, where redevelopment or expansion may be complicated by possible environmental contamination. Contaminants include hazardous waste and/or petroleum.

2. The woman living at 40 Broad Street (Sarah Lewis, wife of police constable Thomas Lewis) lost both her five-month old child, Frances, and husband to cholera. In the four to five day interval between her child's onset of diarrhea on August 28–29, 1854 and subsequent death on September 2, 1854, Mrs. Lewis had soaked the diarrhea-soiled diapers in pails of water. Thereafter she emptied the pails in the cesspool opening in front of her house.

3. Holland, P. W. (1986). Statistics and causal inference. *Journal of the American Statistical Association, 81,* 945–970.

4. After Tufte (1997), p. 33.

5. Latin phrase that well-describes this sort of causal fallacy. Literally it means, "After this, therefore because of this."

6. 1962 also marked the last World Series victory for the New York Yankees before a decades-long draught. Could school prayer have had a hand in that as well?

7. Chapter 1, the Most Dangerous Equation in Wainer (2009). De Moivre's equation states that the variability of an average is equal to the variability of the observations that went into computing that average divided by the square root of the number of those observations. Thus if we calculate averages of 100 observations the variation we would see in such averages would be one-tenth what we would see in the original data. Hence the variability of average cancer rates within counties with a thousand inhabitants would jump around a lot more than those of counties with a million. We would expect to see small counties having both the lowest and the highest of cancer rates. Examining New York's cancer maps confirms this expectation.

8. Age-adjusted death rates—shorthand for a statistical method that allows the effective comparison of groups of individuals that differ in their age distributions. For example, if we look at the mortality rates of, say, the states of Maine and South Carolina, we would find that they are lower in South Carolina. But we would also observe that the population of Maine is generally older. Because older people have higher mortality rates a comparison between the two states might mislead us into thinking that the health of the residents of Maine is worse. To adjust for the differences in age distribution we can calculate the mortality rate for each age group in each state, and then calculate the state-wide mortality rate based on a common (e.g. national) age distribution. Such a summary is then referred to as an age-adjusted death rate.

CHAPTER 2

This chapter is based on "A centenary celebration for Will Burtin: A pioneer of scientific visualization", *Chance*, *22*(1), 51–55, 2009 and "Pictures at an exhibition" (with M. Larsen), *Chance*, *22*(2), 46–54, 2009.

1. Wilhelm Burtin (1908–1972), was born in Ehrenfeld, a suburb of Cologne, the only son of August and Gertrude Bürtin. He successfully began his career in Germany, despite the dismal economic conditions in Germany after World War I and the depression. During his career as one of the foremost graphic designers of the 20th century, he had an enormous influence on the character of modern design and, more specifically to the point of this chapter, he was an early developer of what has come to be called scientific visualization.

2. His departure from Germany was also a departure from most things German; he adamantly refused to speak German. In 1946 he visited Albert Einstein as part of the research for a *Fortune* article "The physics of the bomb," which would feature a picture of Einstein on the cover. Einstein was then actively trying to convince the

world of the dangers of nuclear weapons that were not under international control. Einstein would not speak English with Burtin and Burtin would not speak German with Einstein. So the interview was conducted bilingually.

3. In Conan Doyle's Sherlock Holmes mystery *Silver Blaze*, the groom for the famous racehorse Silver Blaze was found bludgeoned to death in a field. When the Scotland Yard detective Gregory asked Holmes "Is there any other point to which you would wish to draw my attention?" the great detective replied, "To the curious incident of the dog in the night-time." Gregory responded, puzzled that, "The dog did nothing in the night-time." Holmes explained, "That was the curious incident."

4. *Aerobacter (Enterobacter) aerogenes*—Accessed from http://www.eletra.com/ pureaircontrols/pureaircontrols_e_a000175899.JPG (December 31, 2008).

Bacillus anthracis—Photomicrograph of *Bacillus anthracis* from an agar culture demonstrating spores; Fuchsin-methylene blue spore stain. Created by the United States Centers for Disease Control and Prevention. Accessed from http://commons. wikimedia.org/wiki/File:Bacillus_anthracis.png (December 31, 2008).

Brucella abortus—Copyright Dennis Kunkel Microscopy, Inc. Accessed from http:// patric.vbi.vt.edu/organism/overview/images/1.jpg (December 31, 2008).

Diplococcus (Streptococcus) pneumoniae—Scanning electron micrograph of *Streptococcus pneumoniae*. From the United States Centers for Disease Control and Prevention Public Health Image Library. Accessed from http://en.wikipedia.org/ wiki/File:Streptococcus_pneumoniae.jpg (December 31, 2008).

Escherichia coli—Accessed from http://www.eadgene.info/Portals/0/Photos/ Salmonella%20source%20NIAID%20from%20wikipedia%20free%20use%20-%20 cropped.jpg (December 31, 2008). Originally obtained from Wikipedia and listed as free use.

Klebsiella pneumoniae—Public domain. Accessed from http://commons.wikimedia. org/wiki/File:Klebsiella-pneumoniae.jpg (December 31, 2008).

Mycobacterium tuberculosis—From the United States Centers for Disease Control and Prevention Public Health Image Library. Accessed from http://commons. wikimedia.org/wiki/File:Mycobacterium_tuberculosis_8438_lores.jpg (December 31, 2008).

Proteus vulgaris—© Copyright by Satoshi Sasayama, PhD. Accessed from http:// en.citizendium.org/wiki/Image:Proteus_vulgaris.jpg (December 31, 2008). Use of this image requires the express written permission of the copyright holder.

Pseudomonas aeruginosa—This colorized version of PHIL 232 depicts a scanning electron micrograph (SEM) of a number of *Pseudomonas aeruginosa* bacteria. From the United States Centers for Disease Control and Prevention Public Health Image Library. Accessed from http://commons.wikimedia.org/wiki/File:Pseudomonas.jpg (December 31, 2008).

Salmonella (Eberthella) typhosa (typhi)—Rocky Mountain Laboratories, NIAID, NIH. A color-enhanced scanning electron micrograph showing *Salmonella typhimurium* (red) invading cultured human cells. http://commons.wikimedia.org/wiki/File:Salmonella_Typhimurium_Invades_Human_Cells.jpg (December 31, 2008).

Salmonella schottmuelleri—Accessed from http://www.ars.usda.gov/IS/espanol/kids/animals/story2/tails.jpg (December 31, 2008).

Staphylococcus albus (epidermidis)—Scanning electron micrograph of *Staphylococcus epidermidis*. From the United States Centers for Disease Control and Prevention Public Health Image Library. Accessed from http://commons.wikimedia.org/wiki/File:Staphylococcus_epidermidis_01.png (December 31, 2008).

Staphylococcus aureus—Bacterial cells of *Staphylococcus aureus*, which is one of the causal agents of mastitis in dairy cows. Its large capsule protects the organism from attack by the cow's immunological defenses. Freeze drying replication, (TEM) Plate #.9513. Accessed from http://emu.arsusda.gov/typesof/pages/staph.html (December 31, 2008).

Streptococcus (Enterococcus) faecalis—Scanning electron micrograph of *Enterococcus faecalis*. From the United States Centers for Disease Control and Prevention Public Health Image Library. Accessed from http://commons.wikimedia.org/wiki/File:Enterococcus_faecalis_SEM_01.png (December 31, 2008).

Streptococcus hemolyticus—Photomicrograph of *Streptococcus pyogenes* bacteria, 900x Mag. A pus specimen, viewed using Pappenheim's stain. Note *Streptococcus pygenes* is beta-haemolytic. From the United States Centers for Disease Control and Prevention Public Health Image Library. Accessed from http://en.wikipedia.org/wiki/File:Streptococcus_pyogenes_01.jpg (December 31, 2008).

Streptococcus viridans—"*Streptococcus*" group *viridans* bacteria grown in a blood culture. From the United States Centers for Disease Control and Prevention Public Health Image Library. Accessed from http://commons.wikimedia.org/wiki/File:Streptococcus_viridans_01.png (December 31, 2008).

5. Sometimes authors are confronted with an editorial restriction "to use no more figures than absolutely necessary" although a parallel restriction for unnecessary words is rarely as strident. Yet, who is to say that a figure is not, em-for-em, *more* efficiently communicating quantitative phenomena than prose.

CHAPTER 3

This chapter is based on "That's funny . . . " (with S. Lysen), *The American Scientist, 97* (July–August), 272–275, 2009.

1. The work owes much to my colleagues: to Shaun Lysen who co-authored the original paper from which this chapter was based, to Jana Asher who uncovered the change in classification, to Brian Schmotzer for Figure 3.3, to Steve Clyman, Peter Katsufrakis and Steve Goodman for help in understanding the taxonomy of modern bacteriology, and to Ulana Luciw for her help in surveying the usage of displays in the medical literature.

CHAPTER 4

This chapter is based on "Commentary on the 2008 National Healthcare Quality Report and State Snapshots", *Chance*, *23*(2), 45–51, 2010.

1. Report can be retrieved at: http://www.ahrq.gov/qual/nhqr08/nhqr08.pdf.

2. See Wainer (2005, Chapter 10) for instructions on how to do this and further examples.

3. Linda Pickle's wonderful *Atlas of Mortality* provides an almost flawless model for all such work.

4. Cleveland (1994a; 1994b).

CHAPTER 5

This chapter is based on "Improving graphic displays by controlling creativity (with discussion)", *Chance*, *21*(2), 46–53, 2008.

1. This simple? Reality, as always, was more complicated. A more accurate description would be to keep creativity within prescribed bound—neither too much nor too little. Dr. Pickle wrote, "The challenge at National Center for Health Statistics (NCHS) was not to control rampant creativity, but to encourage some degree of it. NCHS has a long history of producing reports of U.S. health statistics. The staff statisticians take their role of guarding the integrity of the data very seriously. Therefore they preferred to publish tables, from which any question could be accurately answered, rather than graphics from which only an approximation of the original value could be extracted. Similarly, they preferred to keep the formats of the tables constant, year after year, so that, as Howard points out, the user need not learn a new format each year. Thus, the challenge for the Atlas team was to overcome the complaint 'but we've never done it that way before.' Most agreed that the atlases that we had previously published at the National Cancer Institute (NCI) had demonstrated the value of looking for geographic patterns in mortality rates, but were hesitant to try any design deviating from that one, i.e. a red-blue color scheme, rates categorized by a combination of rank and statistical significance, and most areas with non-significant rates blanked out."

2. See Wainer (2005), Chapter 5, for an elaboration.

3. http://progressreport.cancer.gov (This site currently contains the 2011/12 Report.)

4. Moss Hart, voiced his appreciation of the value of collaboration, calling it "geld by association." I agree.

CHAPTER 6

This chapter is based on "Looking at blood sugar" (with P. Velleman), *Chance*, *21*(4), 56–61, 2008.

Early release of 2006 data in Chapter 14 of the National Health Interview Survey data, chapter prepared under the auspices of the Center for Disease Control. Available at http://www.cdc.gov/nchs/data/nhis/earlyrelease/earlyrelease200703.pdf.

1. Data from http://diabetes.niddk.nih.gov/DM/PUBS/statistics/#allages.

2. This chapter grew from an article co-authored with Paul Velleman of Cornell University. I am grateful for his permission to reuse it here.

CHAPTER 7

This chapter is based on 'Hip psychometrics' (with P. Baldwin and J. Bernstein), *Statistics in Medicine*, *28*(17), 2277–2292, 2009.

1. The chapter was drawn from an article co-authored with Peter Baldwin of the National Board of Medical Examiners and Joseph Bernstein from the medical school of The University of Pennsylvania. I am grateful for their permission to reuse this material here.

CHAPTER 8

This chapter is based on "Until proven guilty: False positives and the war on terror" (with S. Savage), *Chance*, *21*(1), 55–58, 2008 and "How should we screen for breast cancer: Using evidence to make medical decisions", *Significance*, *8*(1), 28–30, 2011.

1. This chapter grew from an article co-authored with Sam Savage of Stanford University. I am grateful to Sam for his permission to reuse the material.

2. There is a huge research literature on breast cancer, much of which looks into this very question. But the results vary. One recent study (Berg et al. 2008) found that mammography had an accuracy of 78%, but when combined with ultrasound was boosted to 91%. So the figure that I use of 90% accuracy for mammograms alone does no damage to the reputation of mammography.

3. The analyses I have done are meant to yield rough estimates that can provide enough accuracy to guide policy makers. Others have done more careful analyses. Tabar et al. (2004) studied 77,000 women who were randomly chosen to be offered mammogram screening and compared them with 56,000 women who were not. They found that for every 1,500 mammograms administered they were able to extend one life. Including false positives and costs of biopsies yields an estimated cost not unlike the one in (8.3).

4. September 22, 2010 article in the *The New York Times* entitled "Mammograms' value in cancer fight at issue" written by Gina Kolata.

5. The PSA also yields a substantial proportion of false negatives—men with both prostate cancer and normal PSAs. So all subsequent estimates of the cost of PSAs are conservative and estimates of its efficacy are generous. Consideration of this aspect would only strengthen my argument, which I reckon is strong enough without it—no use beating a dead horse.

6. There are some recent studies published on the PSA test. In a study in the US 77,000 men were split into two groups, one got the PSA test and the other did not. While more cancers were found and treated in the first group, the men in that group did

not live longer. A European study found it took screening 1,410 men and treating 48 of them to lengthen one life.

7. This example has been described earlier in Savage & Wainer (2008) and expanded upon in Savage (2009).

8. This methodology of educated multiple guesswork is sometimes called "multiple imputation." The basic idea is that the magic of modern statistics cannot supply numbers where you have none (e.g. the number of terrorists, the accuracy of secret terrorist detecting software). But what it can do is provide an estimate of the range of values likely with your level of ignorance. So we make up a number that seems plausible and try it out. Then another and try that. We continue imputing various possible numbers until we are convinced that we have spanned the range of plausible values. Then we examine the variability of the outcomes. If, as with terrorists, we find that the minimum number of innocent people incorrectly branded as terrorists is still unconscionably large we can safely reject that strategy as being unworkable.

CHAPTER 9

This chapter is based on "Assessing long-term risk with short-term data" (with L. Hubert), *Significance*, 8(4), 170–171, 2011.

1. This chapter was drawn from a paper co-authored with Lawrence Hubert of University of Illinois. I am grateful for his permission to use it here.

2. One of the drugs was a bisphosphonate, which is widely used to prevent fractures, especially of the hip and spine, common in people with osteoporosis; the second was Avandia, usually prescribed to reduce the risk of heart disease in diabetics, but which apparently increases the risk after long-term use.

3. It is well known that the carcinogenic effect of tobacco takes many years to show up. This explains why, despite many attempts at measuring the causal effect of smoking on laboratory animals, it has never been verified. Dogs don't live long enough and they can't seem to teach tortoises to smoke.

4. In a recent refusal from the FDA (October of 2010), the anti-obesity drug, Lorcaserin, was not approved primarily because of tumor formation in rats when the drug was administered in very high doses. The FDA asked for an independent review of the animal data and new studies to assess how relevant the animal findings were to humans.

5. There are several quantitative phenomena useful in statistical explanation within life-testing but that are less than transparent to understand. One particularly bedeviling result is called the Inspection Paradox. Suppose a light bulb now burning above your desk (with an average rated life of, say, 2,000 hours) has been in operation for a year (over 8,000 hours). It now has an expected life longer than 2,000 hours because it has already been on for a while, and therefore cannot burn out at any earlier time than right now. The same is true for life-spans in general. Because we are not, "dead yet," and we cannot die at any earlier time than right now, our life-spans have an

expectancy longer than what they were when we were born. This is good news brought to you by Probability and Statistics!

CHAPTER 10

This chapter is based on "A remarkable horse: An inquiry into the accuracy of medical predictions" (with L. Hubert), *Chance*, *24*(4), 55–57, 2012.

1. This chapter was extracted from an article that was co-authored with Lawrence Hubert of the University of Illinois. I would like to thank him for his permission to reuse it here.

2. Our thanks to Linda Steinberg for the Samuel Johnson quote, to Charles Lewis for helpful conversations and to Steve Clyman and Peter Scoles for pointing us to the appendicitis example.

3. Friend of the Court.

4. Sir William Blackstone, in his 1765 *Commentary on the Laws of England*, provided a similar view, albeit with a slightly different loss function, when he said that, "It is better that ten guilty persons escape than one innocent suffer."

5. Such complications can be very dangerous and have taken the lives of many. Among these are such luminaries as medicine's Walter Reed, magic's Harry Houdini, and mathematics' Hermann Minkowski.

CHAPTER 11

This chapter is based on "On the role of replication in the advance of science: The survival of the fittest", *The American Scientist*, *100* (September–October), 358–361, 2012.

1. My gratitude to David Donoho who, over dinner one evening, told me about the results of a meta-analysis of Chinese medical research, thus instigating this chapter.

2. For example, if you looked carefully, you could see an outline of the pattern on the ESP test card from their back-side. Such flaws are often overlooked by scientists inexperienced in magic. Stanford statistician and magician Persi Diaconis spent a fair amount of time debunking claims of extrasensory perception made by Uri Geller and others. Diaconis said that he was uniquely qualified for such a task; magicians couldn't do it because they didn't understand experimental design, and psychologists couldn't do it because they didn't know magic. His claim has subsequently been borne out by evidence.

3. Actually, even leeches have found a use in modern medicine that, apparently, is based upon evidence. Specifically, during the process of feeding, leeches secrete a complex mixture of different biologically and pharmacologically active substances into the wound. Hirudin is the best known component of leech saliva and it inhibits blood coagulation. Hence even leeches have proved to be of some limited use in the treatment of inflammatory reactions.

4. A meta-analysis is a study that rigorously combines the findings of many other studies in an effort to establish a more rigorous conclusion based on the totality of what

has been done. A meta-analysis is much more than just a research review, in that it combines results in a rigorous way, allowing each study to be weighted proportional to its validity.

5. The phenotype of an organism is the physical appearance or biochemical characteristics as a result of the interaction of its genes and the environment.

SECTION III

1. Dee Hock is the founder and former CEO of VISA International.

2. Lewicka, M. "Confirmation BIAS: Cognitive error or adaptive strategy of action control?". In Mirosław Kofta, Gifford Weary & Grzegorz Sedek (1998). *Personal Control in Action: Cognitive and Motivational Mechanisms*, Springer, 233–255 and Bensley, D. A. (1998). *Critical Thinking in Psychology: A Unified Skills Approach*, Brooks/Cole, 137.

3. Oswald, M. E. & Grosjean, S. (2004). Confirmation bias. In Pohl, Rüdiger F., *Cognitive Illusions: A Handbook on Fallacies and Biases in Thinking, Judgement and Memory*, Psychology Press, Hove, UK, 79–96.

4. Dorothy Parker concurred, as only she could, with her quip that, "You can't teach an old dogma new tricks."

CHAPTER 12

1. My thanks to Stephen Clyman and Robert Galbraith for their help and advice in the preparation of this chapter. Also much has been taken, often in whole cloth from Atul Gawande's remarkable piece "The Checklist"; all unattributed quotations come from him.

2. Puerperal fever (from the Latin *puer*, male child (boy)), also called childbed fever, can develop into puerperal sepsis, which is a serious form of septicaemia contracted by a woman during or shortly after childbirth, miscarriage or abortion. If untreated, it is life-threatening.

3. All women who came to the hospital for clinic care were assigned to one clinic or the other on alternate days.

4. For example, in 1546 Girolamo Fracastoro (1478–1553) proposed that epidemic diseases were caused by transferable tiny particles or "spores" that could transmit infections.

5. I am reminded of Henny Youngman, who responded to the question, "How's your wife?" with the quip, "Compared to what?"

6. Here the ancient model of the universe comes to mind, in which the Earth is supported on Altas' broad shoulders. The question naturally arises, what is Atlas standing on? The ancients had an answer for this too. Atlas stood atop an enormous tortoise. And what supports the tortoise? Another, even larger tortoise. And after that it was turtles all the way down.

7. An anecdote that, if validated by a more rigorous data gathering effort, is suggestive of a solution. At a local teaching hospital I noted that everyone there was always

washing their hands, whereas at a nearby hospital without students this was not the case. One inference that we might draw is that the doctors at the first hospital feel obligated to follow their own advice while the students are watching, whereas at the second, without the watchful eyes of students, the physicians allow the pressures of their jobs to get in the way.

CHAPTER 13

This chapter is based on "Why is a raven like a writing desk? Musing on the power of convention", *The American Scientist*, *96*, 446–449, 2008.

1. My gratitude to the National Board of Medical Examiners for support of this research, despite its only very marginal relationship to NBME's mission. I appreciate the breadth of their view. I also wish to thank Kyung T. Han for his invaluable help in providing expertise in Hangul so that I have some faith that my description of it is reasonably accurate. My thanks also to Paul Velleman, who showed me how to find both Dvorak and Hangul on my Mac, and to David Hoaglin, whose sharp eyes helped me to say more nearly what I meant.

2. Of course it is impossible to underestimate the graphical skills of the mass media. The graphics experts at Fox News showed that their skills matched those of their news department colleagues when they made a pie whose slices summed to 193%!

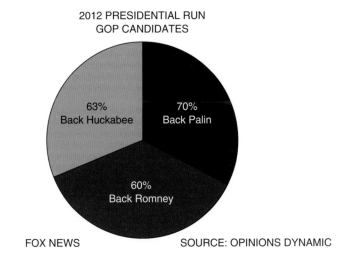

2012 PRESIDENTIAL RUN
GOP CANDIDATES

63%
Back Huckabee

70%
Back Palin

60%
Back Romney

FOX NEWS   SOURCE: OPINIONS DYNAMIC

The news department rose to the challenge by arguing in support of these results (http://flowingdata.com/2009/11/26/fox-news-makes-the-best-pie-chart-ever/).

3. My Macintosh computer has the Dvorak keyboard already built in as an option. It also has the Hangul alphabet.

AFTERWORD

1. 1927–2011, a computer scientist and the father of "Artificial Intelligence."

2. The Catholic Church counts over a billion souls among its members and continues to exist after two millennia and refuses to canonize anyone who is still alive; indeed to become a saint one must not only be dead, but must have been dead for a considerable length of time.

3. From an article by Seth Cline in US News & World Report http://www.usnews.com/news/articles/2012/06/01/sea-level-bill-would-allow-north-carolina-to-stick-its-head-in-the-sand.

4. Actually these three paragraphs were part of an April Fool's joke easily found on the internet http://www.physicsforums.com/archive/index.php/t-159768.html, but the fact that you read this far through it confirms how little faith we have in the wisdom of our brethren. This distrust is likely justified, for indeed there had been a number of attempts around the turn of the 20th century, some only narrowly failing, to redefine π on the basis of criteria unrelated to nature's dictates.

BIBLIOGRAPHY

Ackerknecht, E. H. (1967). *Medicine at the Paris Hospital, 1794–1848*. Baltimore, MD: The Johns Hopkins Press.

American Psychiatric Association Task Force on Clinical Aspects of the Violent Individual (1974). *Clinical Aspects of the Violent Individual*. American Psychiatric Association.

American Cancer Society. http://www.cancer.org.

Andrewes, F. W. & Horder, T. J. (1906). A study of the streptococci pathogenic for man. *Lancet, 2*, 708–713.

Baldwin, P., Bernstein, J. & Wainer, H. (2009). Hip psychometrics. *Statistics in Medicine, 28*, 2277–2292.

Berg, W. A. et al. (2008). Combined screening with ultrasound and mammography vs mammography alone in women at elevated risk of breast cancer. *Journal of the American Medical Association, 299*(18), 2151–2163.

Bertin, J. (1973). *Semiologie Graphique*. The Hague: Mouton-Gautier. 2nd edn. (English translation done by William Berg & Howard Wainer and published as *Semiology of Graphics*, Madison, WI: University of Wisconsin Press, 1983. Latest edition of the English translation published in 2010 by ESRI Press in Redlands, California.)

Bertin, J. (1977). *La graphique et le traitement graphique de l'information*. Paris: Flammarion.

Cleveland, W. S. (1985). *The Elements of Graphing Data*. Boston, MA: Duxbury.

Cleveland, W. S. (1994a). *The Elements of Graphing Data*. Summit, NJ: Hobart Press.

Cleveland, W. S. (1994b). *Visualizing Data*. Summit, NJ: Hobart Press.

Debré, P. & Forster, E. (1998). *Louis Pasteur*. Baltimore, MD: Johns Hopkins University Press.

Diamond Sutra Recitation Group (2004). *King Sejong the Great: The Everlasting Light of Korea*. Seoul, Korea: Diamond Sutra Recitation Group.

Farquhar, A. B. & Farquhar, H. (1891). *Economic and Industrial Delusions: A discourse of the case for protection*. New York: Putnam.

Francis, T. (1955). An evaluation of the 1954 poliomyelitis vaccine trials—summary report. *American Journal of Public Health, 45,* 1–63.

Franklin, R. & Gosling, R. G. (1953). Molecular configuration in sodium thymonucleate. *Nature, 171,* 740–741.

Garden, R. S. (1961). Low-angle fixation in fractures of the femoral neck. *Journal of Bone and Joint Surgery,* 43-B, 647–663.

Gawande, A. (December 10, 2007). The check-list. *The New Yorker.* http://www.newyorker.com/reporting/2007/12/10/071210fa_fact_gawande.

Gelman, A. & Nolan, D. (2002). *Teaching Statistics: A Bag of Tricks.* Oxford: Oxford University Press.

Gøtzsche, P. C. & Nielsen, M. (2009). Screening for breast cancer with mammography. Cochrane Database of Systematic Reviews, Issue 4. Art. No.: CD001877. DOI: 10.1002/14651858.CD001877.pub3. http://www2.cochrane.org/reviews/en/ab001877.html

Graff, L., Russell, J., Seashore, J., Tate, J., Elwell, A., Prete, M., Werdmann, M., Maag, R., Krivenko, C. & Radford, M. (2000). False-negative and false-positive errors in abdominal pain evaluation: failure to diagnose acute appendicitis and unnecessary surgery. *Academy of Emergency Medicine, 7*(11), 1244–1255.

Gregoire, G., Derderian, F. & Le Lorier, J. (1995). Selecting the language of the publications included in a meta-analysis: Is there a Tower of Babel bias? *Journal of Clinical Epidemiology, 48,* 159–163.

Gulliksen, H. O. (1938). Extrasensory perception: What is it? *American Journal of Sociology, 43*(4), 623–634.

Hanninen, O., Farago, M. & Monos, E. (September–October 1983). Ignaz Philipp Semmelweis, the prophet of bacteriology. *Infection Control, 4*(5), 367–370.

Holland, P. W. (1986). Statistics and causal inference. *Journal of the American Statistical Association, 81,* 945–970.

Howard, J. V. & Gooder, H. (1974). Specificity of the autolysin of *Streptococcus (Diplococcus) pneumoniae. Journal of Bacteriology, 117,* 796–804.

Ioannidis, J. P. (August, 2005). Why most published research findings are false. *PLoS Medicine, 2*(8), e124.

Jaynes, J. (1966). The routes of science. *American Scientist, 54*(1), 94–102.

Johnson, S. (2006). *The Ghost Map: The Story of London's most Terrifying Epidemic—and How it Changed Science, Cities, and the Modern World.* New York: Riverhead Books.

Kahneman, D. (2011). *Thinking, Fast and Slow.* New York: Farrar, Straus & Giroux.

Kalager, M., Zelen, M., Langmark, F. & Adami, H. (2010). Effect of screening mammography on breast-cancer mortality in Norway. *New England Journal of Medicine, 363,* 1203–1210.

Kenny, S. J., Aubert, R. E. & Geiss, L. S. (1994). Prevalence and incidence of non-insulin-dependent diabetes. Chapter 4 in *Diabetes in America*. 2nd edn. http://diabetes.niddk.nih.gov/dm/pubs/america

Kolata, G. (September 22, 2010). Mammograms' value in cancer fight at issue. *The New York Times.*

LaPorte, R. E., Matsushima, M. & Chang, Y-F. (1994). Prevalence and incidence of insulin-dependent diabetes. Chapter 3 in *Diabetes in America*. 2nd edn. http://diabetes.niddk.nih.gov/dm/pubs/america

Lehrer, J. (December 13, 2010). The truth wears off: Is there something wrong with the scientific method? *The New Yorker.*

Louis, P. C. A. (1828). Recherche sur les effets de la saignée dans plusieurs maladies inflammatoires. *Archives générales de médecine, 18*, 321–336.

Louis, P. C. A. (1835). *Recherches sur les effets de la saignée dans quelques maladies inflammatoires et sur l'action de l'émétique et des vésicatoires dans la pneumonie.* Paris: Librairie de l'Académie royale de médecine. Republished in English in 1836 as *Researches on the Effects of Bloodletting in Some Inflammatory Diseases.* Boston, MA: Hilliard, Gray and Company.

May, M. T. (translator) (1968). *Galen: On the Usefulness of the Parts of the Body.* Ithaca, NY: Cornell University Press.

Minard, C. J. *Tableaus graphiques et cartes figuratives de M. Minard, 1845–1869.*

Monahan, J. (1981). *The Clinical Prediction of Violent Behavior.* Washington, DC: Government Printing Office.

National Cancer Institute. http://www.cancer.gov/cancertopics/factsheet/detection/PSA.

Nielson, M. (2009). *Screening for Breast Cancer with Mammography: A Review.* New York: John Wiley (from the Cochrane Collaboration http://www.thecochranelibrary.com).

Nielson, M., Thomsen, J. L., Primdahl, S., Dyreborg, U. & Chen, H. H. (1987). Breast cancer and atypia among young and middle-aged women: A study of 110 medicolegal autopsies. *British Journal of Cancer, 56*(6), 814–819.

Nightingale, F. (1858). *Notes on Matters Affecting the Health, Efficiency and Hospital Administration of the British Army.* London: Harrison and Sons.

Nuland, S. B. (2003). *The Doctors' Plague: Germs, Childbed Fever and the Strange Story of Ignac Semmelweis.* New York: W. W. Norton.

Omniglot. http://www.omniglot.com/writing/korean.htm.

Pan, Z., Trikalinos, T. A., Kavvoura, F. K., Lau, J. & Ioannidis, J. (2010). Local literature bias in genetic epidemiology: An empirical evaluation of the Chinese literature. *PLoS Medicine, 7*, e334.

Pickle, L. W. (2008). Commentary on 'Improving graphic displays by controlling creativity'. *Chance, 21*, 53.

Pickle, L. W., Mungiole, M., Jones, G. K. & White, A. A. (1996). *Atlas of United States Mortality*. Hyattsville, MD: National Center for Health Statistics.

Pittet, D. (March–April 2001). Improving adherence to hand hygiene practice: A multidisciplinary approach. *Emerging Infectious Diseases, 7*(2). http://www.cdc.gov/ncidod/ EID/vol7no2/pittet.htm.

Playfair, W. (1786). *The Commercial and Political Atlas*. London: Corry.

Playfair, W. (1801). *The Statistical Breviary*. London: T. Bensley.

Priestley, J. (1765). *A Chart of Biography*. London: William Eyres.

Priestley, J. (1769). *A New Chart of History*. London. Reprinted: 1792, New Haven: Amos Doolittle.

Prostate Cancer Foundation. http://www.prostatecancerfoundation.org.

Remington, R. R. & Fripp, R. S. P. (2007). *Design and Science: The Life and Work of Will Burtin*. Hampshire: Lund Humphries.

Rhine, J. B. (1934). *Extra-Sensory Perception*. Boston, MA: Bruce Humphries.

Saaddine, J. B., Cadwell, B., Gregg, E., Engelgau, M., Vinicor, F., Imperatore, G. and Narayan, V. (2006). Improvements in diabetes processes of care and intermediate outcomes: United States, 1988–2002. *Annals of Internal Medicine, 144*(7), 465–474.

Santayana, G. (1905). *Life of Reason*. Vol. I, Chapter 12. New York: Charles Scribner & Sons.

Saunders, J. B., de C. M. & O'Malley, C. D. (1982). *The Anatomical Drawings of Andreas Vesalius*. New York: Bonanza Books.

Savage, S. (2009). *The Flaw of Averages*. New York: John Wiley.

Savage, S. & Wainer, H. (2008). Until proven guilty: False positives and the war on terror. *Chance, 21*(1), 55–58.

Schleifer, K. H. & Kilpper-Balz, R. (1984). Transfer of *Streptococcus faecalis* and *Streptococcus faecium* to the genus *Enterococcus* nom. rev. as *Enterococcus faecalis* comb. nov. and *Enterococcus faecium* comb. nov. *International Journal of Systemic Bacteriology, 34*, 31–34.

Scope (1951). Neomycin in Skin Infections: A New Topical Antibiotic with a Wide Antibacterial Range and Rarely Sensitizing. *III*(5), 4–7. The Upjohn Company.

Semmelweis, I.; CodellCarter, K. (translator, extensive foreword) (September 15, 1983) [1861] . *Etiology, Concept and Prophylaxis of Childbed Fever*. Madison, WI: University of Wisconsin Press.

Sherman, J. M., Mauer, J. C. & Stark, P. (1937). *Streptococcus fecalis*. *Journal of Bacteriology, 33*(3), 275–282.

Snow, J. (1855). *On the Mode of Communication of Cholera*. London: John Churchill.

Stone, A. (1975). *Mental Health and Law: A System in Transition*. Washington, DC: National Institute of Mental Health.

Tabar, L., Vitak, B., Yen, M. F. A., Chen, H. H. T., Smith, R. A. & Duffy, S. W. (2004). Number needed to screen: Lives saved over 20 years of follow-up in mammographic screening. *Journal of Medical Screening, 11*(3), 126–129.

Taylor, I. (1980). The Korean writing system: An alphabet? A syllabary? A logography? In Kolers, P., Wrolstad, M. E. & Bouma, H. (Eds.). *Processing of Visible Language: 2*. New York: Plenum, 67–82.

Tufte, E. R. (1983). *The Visual Display of Quantitative Information*. Cheshire, CT: Graphics Press.

Tufte, E. R. (1997). *Visual Explanations*. Cheshire, CT: Graphics Press.

Tukey, J. W. (1977). *Exploratory Data Analysis*. Boston, MA: Addison-Wesley.

Van Der Weyden, M. B., Armstrong, R. M. & Gregory, A. T. (2005). The 2005 Nobel Prize in physiology or medicine. *Medical Journal of Australia, 183*(11–12), 612–614.

Wainer, H. (1997). *Visual Revelations: Graphical Tales of Fate and Deception from Napoleon Bonaparte to Ross Perot*. New York: Copernicus Books.

Wainer, H. (2005). *Graphic Discovery: A Trout in the Milk and Other Visual Adventures*. Princeton, NJ: Princeton University Press.

Wainer, H. (2008). Improving graphic displays by controlling creativity. *Chance, 21*, 46–52.

Wainer, H. (2009). *Picturing the Uncertain World: How to Understand, Communicate and Control Uncertainty through Graphical Display*. Princeton, NJ: Princeton University Press.

Wainer, H., Bradlow, E. T. & Wang, X. (2007). *Testlet Response Theory and its Applications*. New York: Cambridge University Press.

Watson, J. D. & Crick, F. H. C. (1953). Genetical implications of the structure of deoxyribose nucleic acid. *Nature, 171*, 964–967.

Watson, J. D. & Crick, F. H. C. (1953). A structure for deoxyribose nucleic acid. *Nature, 171*, 737–738.

Wikipedia. http://en.wikipedia.org/wiki/Hangul#History

Wilkins, M. H. F., Stokes, A. R. & Wilson, H. R. (1953). Molecular structure of deoxyribose nucleic acid. *Nature, 171*, 738–740.

Wurman, S. (Ed.) (2000). *Understanding USA*. New York: Markle Foundation.

INDEX

A

accelerated life testing 120–1,
    161–2
airplanes, checklists for
    flying 136–7
Albee, Edward 155
Allen, Woody vii
ALL, special representation of 61,
    63–7, 83
alphabets, power of convention
    and 147–50, 151
animal experimentation, low-dose
    extrapolation 118–20, 161
antibiotics' impact (on different
    bacteria)
    Burtin's findings and display
        23–9, 50–2
    chapter notes 156–8
    conclusion 47–8
    factors for consideration in data
        display 29–32
    fifteen different data
        displays 32–47, 157–8
    graphic display's role in revealing
        the unexpected xiii–xiv, 8,
        50–8, 158
    introduction to xiii–xiv, 4, 8,
        21–3, 156
appendicitis, error rates in
    suspected 125–6, 162
archiving, as purpose of graphic
    displays 60–1
Asher, Jana viii, 33
Asherman, Georgette viii, 44
Asimov, Isaac xiii, 50
Atlas 163

Atlas of United States Mortality,
    The xiv, 8, 74–8, 159
Australian Medical Journal 143
authority, power of 1, 2, 56, 155
authors, cooperation between 84
Avandia, safety of 118, 161
axis labeling 62, 64, 66, 83

B

Bacon, Francis 56, 127
bacteria
    antibiotics' impact on, *see*
        antibiotics' impact (on
        different bacteria)
    errors in taxonomy 27, 45, 53–8
Baldwin, Peter viii
bar charts
    antibiotics' impact study data
        display 37–9, 42, 45, 53, 54
    dot chart as replacement
        for 39–40, 63–4, 73
    Joseph Priestley's chart of
        biography 78, 79
    *National Healthcare Quality
        Report* (2008) examples/
        suggestions 60–7, 73
Barefoot v. Estelle 122–3
Bernstein, Joseph viii
Bertin, Jacques viii, 52–3
biopsy, cost of cancer detection
    107–8, 111–12, 160
biphosphonates, drug safety 161
Blackstone, Sir William 162
bloodletting 4, 129, 155, 162
blood sugar monitoring, *see*
    glucose meters (data

    summary/display
        improvements)
Boeing's Model 299, checklist use
    135
Brandt, Troy viii, 34
breast cancer
    false positives in mammograms
        106–9, 153, 160
    radiation therapy utilization
        65–6
Brodsky, Richard xiii, 4, 10, 18
brownfields 10, 155
Burtin (Will) viii, xiii, 4, 8, 21–2,
    156–7
    antibiotics' impact study, *see*
        antibiotics' impact (on
        different bacteria)
    cell structure research 22–3

C

calculation, purpose of
    graphs 29
cancer incidence maps
    age adjusted kidney cancer
        rates 16–18
    New York, *see* New York's cancer
        maps
cancer screening, false positives
    in 105–12, 116, 160–1
Cancer Trends Report 81–3
canonization 165
captions 61, 68–9
carcinogenic effect, determination
    of 118–20, 161
car door hinges, accelerated life
    testing 121

causal inferences 11–16, 155–6
cell structure 22–3
Challenger space shuttle 153–4
Chance 29
change
 in medical practice
  chapter notes 163–4
  checklists and medical care
   136–9
  handwashing 139–44
  introduction to xv, 134,
   135–6
  suggestions for future 143–4
 power of convention and
  resistance to xv, 134,
  145–51
Chang, Mindy viii, 39
Chase, Editha viii
checklists, use of 135–8, 141, 143,
 144, 163
China
 language and power of
  convention 148, 150, 151
 replication in medical
  research 130–1
cholera, John Snow's map of
 11–14, 155
choropleth maps 60–1, 71–3
classification
 errors in bacterial 27, 45, 53–8
 of hip fractures 100–3
Clauser, Brian viii
Cleveland, William 146–7, 151
clinical trials, long-term risk
 assessment with shorter-term
 data 117–21, 161–2
Clyman, Steve viii
Cochrane Collaboration 129
coherence, in data display
 30–1, 84
color
 in choropleth maps 71–3
 in line charts 82
colorectal cancer
 death rates 69–71
 screening 67, 72
communication
 contents/introduction of Section
  I (Communicating with the
  Public) xiii–xiv, 7–8
 of diabetic treatment/behavior
  consequences 87–9, 98
 public participation and 7–8

as purpose of graphic display 29,
 30, 32, 61, 152–3
confirmation bias 133, 163
convention, power of xv, 134,
 145–51, 164
cooperation
 among authors 84
 between physician and diabetic
  patients 88
 public 1–2
cost, of false positives in
 detection 107–8, 109,
 111–12, 116
county population, effect on cancer
 incidence maps 16–20
creativity, graphic display
 improvement by
 controlling xiv, 8, 74–84, 159
Crick, F.H.C. 22–3
criminals
 false positives in detection
  of 114–16
 prediction of 'future
  dangerousness' 122–6

D

Dangauthier, Pierre viii, 36
Dartois, Céline viii, 41
data storage 60–1
Da Vinci, Leonardo 2, 3
death rates
 age-adjusted 16–18, 75–8, 156
 colorectal cancer 69–71
 firearm suicide 75–8
 handwashing and maternal
  mortality 139–41
decoration, as graph's purpose 29,
 32–4
Delaney Clause research 118–20
de Moivre's equation 16, 18, 156
detection schemes
 false negatives in 105, 115
 false positives in, *see* false
  positives
Deutsch, David 132
diabetes
 glucose meter improvements,
  see glucose meters
  (data summary/display
  improvements)
 prevalence of 87–8
Diaconis, Persi 162

diagnostic accuracy
 appendicitis (suspected) 125–6,
  162
 confirmation bias and 133
 hip fractures and second
  opinions xiv, 85, 99–104,
  160
Diplococcus pneumoniae, incorrect
 classification of 45, 53–8
DNA
 criminal detection role 114
 structure of 22–3
Donoho, David viii
dot charts/plots
 antibiotics' impact study data
  display 39–40
 as bar chart replacement 39–40,
  63–4, 73
 connecting the dots 41
 frequency of different graphic
  forms 57
 *National Healthcare Quality
  Report* (2008) suggestions
  63–4, 73
 as pie chart replacement 146–7,
  151
Drimmer, Marc ix
drug safety, long-term risk
 assessment with shorter-term
 data 117–21, 161–2
Dultz, Rachel ix
Dvorak, August 151, 164

E

editors
 editorial restriction 158
 leadership from 84
Einstein, Albert 134, 152, 156–7
Emerging Infectious Diseases 141
Enterococcus faecalis, classification
 of 53–8
error rates
 false negatives 105, 115, 125–6
 false positives, *see* false positives
evidence
 change in practice and vii
 definition of 47
 graphic display's role in
  understanding viii, 154
 public cooperation and 1–2
 public participation and
  requirement of 7–8

Evidence-Based Medicine Working Group 1–2
evidence-based science
  historical context of 2–4, 56–7
  meaning of 56
  reasons for slow adoption 133–4
exercise, in diabetes 88, 95–8
exploration, as graph's purpose 29, 32
extrapolation
  in accelerated life testing 120–1
  line charts and linear 69–71
  low-dose 118–20, 121
extra-sensory perception (ESP), study on 128, 162

F

faith 56
false negatives 105, 115, 125–6
false positives
  conclusion on 116
  in detection of criminals 114–15
  in 'future dangerousness' prediction 124–6
  introduction to xv, 85–6, 105, 160
  in mammograms 106–9, 153, 160
  in prostate-specific antigen (PSA) test 110–12, 160–1
  scientific tolerance of 127–8
  in wiretaps for terrorist detection 112–14, 161
Feynman, Richard P. 153–4
financial incentives, for practice change 138, 144
Finer, Lawrence B. viii, 36
font 83
food additives, carcinogenic effect determination 118–20, 161
Fortune 156–7
Fracastoro, Girolamo 163
'future dangerousness', prediction of 122–6

G

Galbraith, Bob viii
Galen of Pergamum, the uterus 2–3
garbage, contents of New York City's 146–7
Garden classification, hip fracture 100–3
gastritis, practice change 143–4

Gawande, Atul 136, 141, 163
glucose meters (data summary/display improvements)
  chapter notes 159–60
  conclusions 97–8
  current functions 89
  example 94–7
  introduction xiv, 85, 87–9
  suggestions for 89–93
Gram staining 24
  antibiotics' impact and, *see* antibiotics' impact (on different bacteria)
graphic displays
  communication of antibiotics' impact study findings, *see* antibiotics' impact (on different bacteria)
  National Healthcare Quality Report (2008) suggestions, *see National Healthcare Quality Report* (NHQR) (2008)
  purpose and important features of 29–32, 60–1
  role in revealing the unexpected 50–8, 158
  theme of this book 152–3
  see also specific features/formats
grid lines 83
Grigson, James 123
Gulliksen, Harold 128

H

Haldar, Dibyojyoti viii, 43
hand washing, increasing compliance 139–43, 144, 163–4
Hangul alphabet, power of convention and 147–50, 151, 164
Han, Kyung viii
healthcare efficacy
  measurement of 59–60, 73
  National Healthcare Quality Report, see *National Healthcare Quality Report* (NHQR) (2008)
Helicobacter pylori 143–4
Helvetica font 83
hip fractures, second opinions xiv, 85, 99–104, 160

historical context, evidence-based medicine/science 2–4, 56–7
Hoaglin, David viii
Hock, Dee 133, 163
horizontal/vertical orientation, of display 63, 64
hybrid displays 34–5

I

icons, in data display 42, 44–7, 53, 54
illumination, as theme of this book 152–4
infection
  antibiotics' impact on, *see* antibiotics' impact (on different bacteria)
  hand washing compliance and 139–44, 163–4
  intravenous line insertion checklists and 137–8
innovation, control of 74–84
inspection paradox 161–2
intensive-care medicine, checklist usage 137–8
intravenous line infection, insertion checklist usage 137–8
Ioanndis, John 128–9

J

Jacobs, Brad 135
Jaynes, Julian 132
Johnson, Samuel 56, 122
Journal of the American Medical Association 1–2, 57

K

Kahneman, Daniel 128
keyboards, power of convention and 145–6, 147, 151, 164
Keystone Initiative 138
kidney cancer, age-adjusted death rates 16–18
Kolata, Gina 117–18, 160
Kollestschka, Jakob 140
Korean language, power of convention and 147–50, 151, 164

L

labeling
  antibiotics' impact study data
    display 42, 43
  line chart suggestions 82, 83
  *National Healthcare Quality
    Report* (2008) improvements
    61, 62–3, 64, 65–6, 68–9
language, power of convention
  and 147–50, 151
Larsen, Michael viii
Lauderdale, Benjamin viii, 35
Lauderdale, Katherine viii, 35
Lawson, Leonard Lee 154
leeches, bloodletting 4, 129, 155,
  162
legends 61, 66–8
Lehrer, Jonah 128–9
Libous, Tom 10, 18
life expectancy 161–2
life testing, accelerated 120–1,
  161–2
light bulbs, accelerated life testing
  120–1, 161–2
line charts
  antibiotics' impact study data
    display 32, 33, 41, 43
  Cancer Trends Report example/
    suggested improvements
    81–3
  linear extrapolation in 69–71
  *National Healthcare Quality
    Report* (2008) examples/
    improvements 60–1, 65–71
Linzmayer, Adam 128
log scales 32, 36, 37, 39, 43, 44
Lorcaserin, safety of 161
Louis, P.C.A. 155
low-dose extrapolation 118–20, 121
Lutz, Brobson 142
Lykoudis, John 143
Lysen, Shaun viii, 55

M

Maimonides, Moses 125, 152
mammograms, false positives in
  106–9, 153, 160
Manli, Choi 150
maps
  *Atlas of United States Mortality,
    The* xiv, 8, 74–8, 159
  choropleth 60–1, 71–3

John Snow's map of cholera
    11–14, 155
  New York's cancer maps, *see*
    New York's cancer maps
Marshall, Barry 143–4
maternal mortality rate, and hand
  washing in 19th century
  139–41
McCarthy, John 153, 165
mean 90–1
  running 92, 93
median, resistant methods 90–1
Melnick, Donald viii
memorability, of data display
  30–1, 34
meta-analysis 131, 162–3
methicillin-resistant *Staphylococcus
  aureus* (MRSA) 142
Mill, John Stuart 134
Minard, Charles Joseph 30–2, 83–4
Monroe, Miles vii
moving average (running mean)
  92, 93
multiple imputation 161
multiples, small 42, 44–5

N

Napoleon, plot of failed Russian
  campaign 30–2
National Healthcare Quality Report
  (NHQR) (2008)
  background information xiv,
    59–60, 159
  discussion and conclusions 73
  examples and suggested
    improvements 62–73
  general display characteristics
    60–62
Nature 22–3
negatives, false 105, 115, 125–6
Neomycin, impact on different
  bacteria, *see* antibiotics'
  impact (on different bacteria)
New England Journal of Medicine
  109, 138
New Yorker, The 128, 135–6
New York's cancer maps
  chapter notes 155–6
  danger of statistical ignorance
    16–20
  identifying SAT score decline
    causation 14–16
  introduction xiii, 4, 8, 10–11

John Snow's map of cholera
    11–14
  Texas Sharpshooter legend
    9–10, 20
New York Times, The vii, xiii, 10,
  117, 146, 160
Nicolich, Mark viii, 46
Nietzsche, Fredrick 135
non-Hodgkin's lymphoma,
  incidence maps 18–20
Nungester, Ron viii

O

obesity
  anti-obesity drug safety 161
  diabetes and xiv, 85, 88, 94–8,
    159–60
opinions, second xiv, 85, 99–104,
  160
ordering 61, 63, 64, 71–3

P

Pan, Zhenglun 131
Pasteur, Louis 140–1
Pearce, Hubert 128
Penicillin, impact on different
  bacteria, *see* antibiotics'
  impact (on different bacteria)
peptic ulcer treatment, practice
  change 143–4
physical exams, evidence
  against vii
pi (π), value of 154, 165
Pickle, Linda 74–5, 159
pie charts, power of convention
  and 146–7, 151, 164
pilots (airplane), checklist usage
  136–7
Piskorowski, Tom 138
Pittet, Didier 141–2
Playfair, William 146
plotting points, deletion of 83
polio, Salk vaccine experiment 7–8
polygons 45–7
population, cancer incidence maps
  and county 16–20
positives, false, *see* false positives
practice, change in, *see* change,
  in medical practice
prayer ban, SAT score decline
  and 14–15
predictions 86